MEDICAL ABBREVIATIONS:

7000 Conveniences at the Expense of Communications and Safety

Fifth Edition, Revised

Neil M. Davis, M.S., Pharm.D., FASHP
Professor of Pharmacy, Temple University
School of Pharmacy, Philadelphia, PA,
Editor-in-Chief, Hospital Pharmacy

published by

Neil M. Davis Associates
1143 Wright Drive
Huntingdon Valley, PA 19006
Phone (215) 947-1752
FAX (215) 938-1937

First edition, 1983, titled, "1700 Medical Abbreviations: Convenience at the Expense of Communications and Safety"

Second edition, 1985, titled, "Medical Abbreviations: 2300 Conveniences at the Expense of Communications and Safety"

Third edition, 1987, titled, "Medical Abbreviations: 4200 Conveniences at the Expense of Communications and Safety"

Fourth edition, 1988, titled, "Medical Abbreviations: 5500 Conveniences at the Expense of Communications and Safety"

Library of Congress Catalog Card Number 90-092957

ISBN 0-931431-05-0

The user must exercise care in that the meaning shown in this book may not be the one intended by a writer. When there is doubt, the writer must be contacted for clarification.

Printed in Canada.

Preface

Listed are 7000 current acronyms, symbols, and other abbreviations and over 11,000 of their possible meanings. This list has been compiled to assist individuals in reading medical records, medically related communications, and prescriptions. The list, although current and comprehensive, represents only a portion of abbreviations in use and their many possible meanings as new ones are being coined every day.

Abbreviations are a convenience, a time saver, a space saver, and a way of avoiding the possibility of misspelling words. However, a price can be paid for their use. Abbreviations are sometimes not understood or are interpreted incorrectly. Their use may lengthen the time needed to train individuals in the health fields, at times delays the patient's care, and occasionally results in patient harm.

The publication of this list of abbreviations is not an endorsement of their legitimacy. It is not a guarantee that the intended meaning has been correctly captured, or an indication that they are in common use. Where uncertainty exists, the one who wrote the abbreviation must be contacted for clarification.

There are many variations in how an abbreviation can be expressed. Anterior-posterior has been written as AP, A.P., ap, and A/P. Since there are few standards and those who use abbreviations do not necessarily follow these standards, this book only shows Anterior-posterior as AP. This is done to make it easier to find the meaning of an abbreviation as all the meanings of APs are listed together. This elimination of unnecessary duplication also keeps the book at a convenient size thus enabling it to be sold at a reasonable price.

The Council of Biology Editors (CBE), in their CBE Style Manual[1], lists about 600 abbreviations gathered from 15 internationally recognized authorities and organizations. The majority of these symbols and abbreviations tend to be more scientifically oriented than those which would appear in medical records. In the few situations where the CBE abbreviations differ from what is presented in this book, the CBE abbreviation has been placed in parenthesis after the meaning. As is the practice in the United States, mL has been used rather than ml and the spelling of liter, meter, etc. is used rather than litre and metre, even though ml, litre, and metre are listed in the CBE Style Manual.

The abbreviation AP, is listed as meaning doxorubicin and cisplatin. The reason for this apparent disparity is that the official generic names, (United States Adopted Names) are shown, rather than the trade names Adriamycin® and Platinol®. In the case of LSD, the official name, lysergide is given, rather than the chemical name, lysergic acid diethylamide. The Latin derivations for older medical and pharmaceutical abbreviations, (TID, *ter in die,* three times daily) may be found in Remington.[2]

Healthcare organizations are wisely required by the Joint Commission on Accreditation of Healthcare Organizations to formulate an approved list of abbreviations. Every attempt should be made to restrict this list to common abbreviations that are understood by all health professionals who must work with medical records. There are certain dangerous abbreviations that should not be approved, and a warning should be issued about their use (See Table 1 as well as notes in the text).

Many inherent problems associated with abbreviations contribute to or cause errors. Reports of such errors have been published routinely.[3-5]

Abbreviations and symbols can also easily be misread or interpreted in a manner not intended. For example:

(1) "HCT250 mg" was intended to mean hydrocortisone 250 mg but was interpreted as hydrochlorothiazide 50 mg (HCTZ50 mg).

(2) Flucytosine was improperly abbreviated as 5 FU causing it to be read as fluorouracil. Flucytosine is abbreviated 5 FC and fluorouracil is 5 FU.

(3) Floxuridine was improperly abbreviated as 5 FU causing it to be read as fluorouracil. Flucytosine is abbreviated FUDR and fluorouracil is 5 FU.

(4) MTX was thought to be mustargen. MTX is methotrexate and mustargen is abbreviated HN_2.

Table 1. Some dangerous abbreviations

Problem term	Reason	Suggested term
O.D. for once daily	Interpreted as right eye	Write "once daily"
q.o.d. for every other day	Interpreted as meaning once daily or read as q.i.d.	Write "every other day"
q.d. for once daily	Read or interpreted as q.i.d.	Write "once daily"
q.n. for every night	Read as every hour	Write "every night," "H.S." or nightly
q hs for every night	Read as every hour	Use "HS" or "at bedtime"
U for Unit	Read as 0, 4 6 or cc.	Write "unit"
O.J. for orange juice	Read as OD or OS	Write "orange juice"
µg (microgram)	When handwritten, misread as mg	Write "mcg"
sq or sub q for subcutaneous	The q is read as every	Use "subcut"
Chemical symbols	Not understood or misunderstood	Write full name
Lettered abbreviations for drug names	Not understood or misunderstood	Use generic or trade name
Apothecary symbols or terms	Not understood or misunderstood	Use metric system
per os for by mouth	OS read as left eye	Use "by mouth," "orally," or "P.O."
D/C for discharge	Interpreted as discontinue (orders for discharge medications result in premature discontinuance of current medication)	Write "discharge"
T/d for one per day	Read as T.I.D.	Use "once daily"
/ (a slash mark) for with, and, or per	read as a one	use, "and", "with", or "per"

(5) **The abbreviation "U" for unit is the most dangerous one in the book, having caused numerous 10 fold insulin overdoses. The word unit should never be abbreviated.** The handwritten U for unit has been mistaken for a zero, causing tenfold errors. The handwritten U has also been read as the number four and as "cc".

(6) OD meant to signify once daily has caused Lugol's solution to be given in the right eye.

(7) OJ meant to signify orange juice, looked like OS and caused Saturated Solution of Potassium Iodide to be given in the left eye.

(8) Na Warfarin (Sodium Warfarin) was read as "No Warfarin."

(9) The abbreviation "s" for without has been thought to mean "with" (c).

(10) The order for PT, intended to signify a laboratory test order for prothrombin time, resulted in the ordering of a physical therapy consultation.

(11) The abbreviation, "TAB", meant to signify Triple Antibiotic, (a coined name for a hospital sterile topical antibiotic mixture), caused patients to have their wound irrigated with a diet soda.

(12) a slash mark (/) has been mistaken for a one causing a patient to receive a 100 unit overdose of NPH insulin when the slash was used to separate an order for two insulin doses.

6 units regular insulin/20 units NPH insulin

A prescription could be written with directions as follows: "OD OD OD," to mean one drop in the right eye once daily!

Abbreviations should not be used for drug names as they are particularly dangerous. As previously illustrated there is the possibility that the writer may, through mental error, confuse two abbreviations and use the wrong one. Similarly, the reader may attribute the wrong meaning to an abbreviation. To further confound the problem, some drug name abbreviations have multiple meanings (see CPM, CPZ and PBZ in table 2). The abbreviation AC has been used for three different cancer chemotherapy

Table 2. Example of abbreviations which have several meanings.

CPM	= cyclophosphamide; chlorpheniramine maleate; continuous passive motion; continue present management; central pontine myelinolysis; counts per minute and clinical practice model
PBZ	= phenylbutazone; pyribenzamine; phenoxybenzamine
CPZ	= chlorpromazine; Compazine®
DW	= dextrose in water; distilled water; deionized water
MS	= morphine sulfate; multiple sclerosis; mitral stenosis; musculoskeletal; medical student; minimal support; muscle strength; mental status; milk shake; mitral sound and morning stiffness
CF	= cystic fibrosis; Caucasian female; calcium leucovorin (citrovorum factor); complement fixation; cancer-free; cardiac failure; coronary flow; contractile force; cephalothin; Christmas factor; count fingers and cisplatin and fluorouracil
NBM	= no bowel movement; normal bowel movement; nothing by mouth; normal bone marrow

combinations to mean, Adriamycin® and either cyclophosphamide, carmustine, or cisplatin. Beside causing medication errors and incorrect interpretation of medical records, abbreviations can create problems because treatment is delayed while a health professional seeks clarification for the meaning of the abbreviation used. Abbreviations should not be used to designate drugs or combinations of drugs.

Certain abbreviations in the book are followed by a warning, "this is a dangerous abbreviation". This warning could be placed after most abbreviations, but was reserved for situations where errors have been published because these abbreviations were used or where the meaning is critical and not likely to be known. Such warning statements should also appear after every abbreviation for a drug or drug combination.

Abbreviations for medical facility names create problems as they are usually not recognized by the reader in another geographic area. A clue to the fact that one is dealing with such an abbreviation is when it ends with MC, for Medical Center: MH, for Memorial Hospital: CH, for Community Hospital: UH, for University Hospital: and H, for Hospital.

When an abbreviation can not be found in the book or when the listed meaning(s) do not make sense, there is a possibility that the abbreviation has been misread. As an example, a reader could not find the meaning of HHTS. On closer examination it really was +HTS, not HHTS.

An examination of the following list is a testimonial to the problems and dangers associated with most undefined abbreviations.

The assistance of Aphirudee Poshakrishma Hemachudha, former teaching assistant, Temple University School of Pharmacy, Philadelphia, PA; Michael R. Cohen, Director of Pharmacy Service, Quakertown Community Hospital, Quakertown, PA; Ann Sandt Kishbaugh, Merchantville, NJ and all the others that helped is gratefully acknowledged.

A

A	accommodation age alive ambulatory angioplasty anterior apical arterial artery assessment
(a)	axillary temperature
ā	before
A_2	aortic second sound
A250	5% albumin 250 mL
A1000	5% albumin 1000 mL
A II	angiotensin II
AA	acetic acid achievement age active assistive Alcoholics Anonymous alcohol abuse alveolar-arterial gradient amino acid antiarrhythmic agent aortic aneurysm aplastic anemia arm ankle (pulse ratio) ascending aorta audiologic assessment authorized absence automobile accident cytarabine and doxorubicin
aa	of each
A&A	arthroscopy and arthrotomy awake and aware
AAA	abdominal aortic aneurysmectomy (aneurysm) acute anxiety attack
AAC	antimicrobial agent-associated colitis
AACG	acute angle closure glaucoma
AAD	acid-ash diet antibiotic associated diarrhea
AAE	active assistance exercise acute allergic encephalitis
A/AEX	active assistive exercise
AAG	alpha-1-acid glycoprotein
AAL	anterior axillary line
AAMS	acute aseptic meningitis syndrome
AAN	analgesic abuse nephropathy analgesic-associated nephropathy attending's admission notes
AAO	alert, awake, & oriented
AAO × 3	awake and oriented to time, place, and person
AAP	assessment adjustment pass
AAPC	antibiotic acquired pseudomembranous colitis
AAPMC	antibiotic-associated pseudomembranous colitis
AAROM	active assistive range of motion
AAS	atlantoaxis subluxation atypical absence seizure
AASCRN	amino acid screen
AAU	acute anterior uveitis
AAV	adeno-associated virus
AAVV	accumulated alveolar ventilatory volume
AB	abortion ace bandage antibiotic antibody
A/B	acid-base ratio apnea/bradycardia
A > B	air greater than bone (conduction)
A & B	apnea and bradycardia
ABC	absolute band counts absolute basophil count apnea, bradycardia, and cyanosis aspiration, biopsy and cytology artificial beta cells

ABCDE	botulism toxoid pentavalent
ABD	after bronchodilator
ABd	plain gauze dressing, type of
Abd	abdomen
	abdominal
	abductor
ABDCT	atrial bolus dynamic computer tomography
ABE	acute bacterial endocarditis
	adult basic education
	botulism equine trivalent antitoxin
ABEP	auditory brainstem-evoked potentials
ABG	aortoiliac bypass graft
	arterial blood gases
	axiobuccogingival
ABI	atherothrombotic brain infarction
ABID	antibody identification
ABK	aphakic bullous keratopathy
ABL	allograft bound lymphocytes
ABLB	alternate binaural loudness balance
A/B Mods	apnea/bradycardia moderate stimulation
A/B MS	apnea/bradycardia mild stimulation
ABMT	autologous bone marrow transplantation
ABN	abnormality(ies)
A.B.N.M.	American Board of Nuclear Medicine
abnor.	abnormal
ABO	blood group system (A, AB B, and O)
ABP	arterial blood pressure
ABR	absolute bed rest
	auditory brain (evoked) responses
ABS	absent
	absorbed
	absorption
	acute brain syndrome
	admitting blood sugar
	at bedside

A/B SS	apnea/bradycardia self-stimulation
ABT	aminopyrine breath test
ABVD	adriamycin, bleomycin, vinblastine, and dacarbazine (DTIC)
ABW	actual body weight
ABx	antibiotics
AC	abdominal circumference
	acetate
	acromioclavicular
	acute
	air conditioned
	air conduction
	anchored catheter
	antecubital
	anticoagulant
	assist control
	before meals
A/C	anterior chamber of the eye
	assist/control
5-AC	azacitidine
ACA	acyclovir
	adenocarcinoma
	aminocaproic acid
	anterior cerebral artery
	anterior communicating artery
AC/A	accommodation convergence–accommodation (ratio)
ACB	alveolar-capillary block
	antibody-coated bacteria
AC & BC	air and bone conduction
ACBE	air contrast barium enema
ACC	accident
	accommodation
	adenoid cystic carcinomas
	administrative control center
	ambulatory care center
AcCoA	acetyl-coenzyme A
ACCR	amylase creatinine clearance ratio
ACD	absolute cardiac dullness
	acid-citrate-dextrose
	anterior chamber diameter
	anterior chest diameter
	dactinomycin
ACDs	anticonvulsant drugs

ACE	angiotensin-converting enzyme
ACF	accessory clinical findings
	acute care facility
ACG	angiocardiography
ACH	adrenal cortical hormone
	aftercoming head
	arm girth, chest depth, and hip width
ACh	acetylcholine
AChE	acetylcholinesterase
AC & HS	before meals and at bedtime
ACI	adrenal cortical insufficiency
	aftercare instructions
ACL	anterior cruciate ligament
ACLS	advanced cardiac life support
ACMV	assist-controlled mechanical ventilation
ACN	acute conditioned neurosis
ACP	acid phosphatase
ACPA	anticytoplasmic antibodies
AC-PH	acid phosphatase
ACPP	adrenocorticopolypeptide
ACPP PF	acid phosphatase prostatic fluid
ACR	adenomatosis of the colon and rectum
	anticonstipation regimen
ACS	American Cancer Society
	anodal-closing sound
ACSVBG	aortocoronary saphenous vein bypass graft
ACSW	Academy of Certified Social Workers
ACT	activated clotting time
	allergen challenge test
	anticoagulant therapy
ACT-D	dactinomycin
Act Ex	active exercise
ACTH	corticotropin (adrenocorticotrophic hormone)
ACTSEB	anterior chamber tube shunt encircling band
ACV	acyclovir
	atrial/carotid/ventricular
ACVD	acute cardiovascular disease
AD	accident dispensary
	admitting diagnosis
	alternating days (this is a dangerous abbreviation)
	Alzheimer's disease
	axis deviation
	right ear
A&D	alcohol and drug
	ascending and descending
	vitamins A and D
ADA	adenosine deaminase
	American Diabetes Association
	anterior descending artery
ADAU	adolescent drug abuse unit
ADC	Aid to Dependent Children
	anxiety disorder clinic
ADCC	antibody-dependent cellular cytotoxicity
ADD	adduction
	attention deficit disorder
	average daily dose
ADDH	attention deficit disorder with hyperactivity
ADDU	alcohol and drug dependence unit
ADE	acute disseminated encephalitis
ADEM	acute disseminating encephalomyelitis
ADFU	agar diffusion for fungus
ADG	atrial diastolic gallop
ADH	antidiuretic hormone
ADI	allowable daily intake
A-DIC	doxorubicin and dacarbazine
ADL	activities of daily living
ad lib	as desired
	at liberty
ADM	admission
	doxorubicin
Ad-OAP	doxorubicin, vincristine, cytarabine, and prednisone
adol	adolescent
ADP	arterial demand pacing
	adenosine diphosphate
ADPKD	autosomal dominant

polycystic kidney disease

ADQ abductor digiti quinti
adequate

ADR acute dystonic reaction
adverse drug reaction
doxorubicin (Adriamycin®)

ADRIA doxorubicin (Adriamycin®)

ADS anatomical dead space
anonymous donor's sperm
antibody deficiency syndrome

ADSU ambulatory diagnostic surgery unit

ADT alternate-day therapy
anticipate discharge tomorrow
Auditory Discrimination Test

ADTP Adolescent Day Treatment Program

A5D5W alcohol 5%, dextrose 5% in water for injection

AE above elbow (amputation)
accident and emergency (department)
air entry
aryepiglottic (fold)

A&E accident and emergency (department)

AEA above elbow amputation

AEB as evidenced by

AEC at earliest convenience

AED antiepileptic drug
automated external defibrillator

AEDP automated external defibrillator pacemaker

AEEU admission entrance and evaluation unit

AEG air encephalogram

AEM ambulatory electrogram monitor

AEq age equivalent

AER acoustic evoked response
auditory evoked response

Aer. M. aerosol mask

Aer. T. aerosol tent

AES anti-embolic stockings

AET atrial ectopic tachycardia

AF acid-fast
amniotic fluid
anterior fontanel
antifibrinogen
aortofemoral
atrial fibrillation

AFB acid-fast bacilli
aorto-femoral bypass
aspirated foreign body

AFBG aortofemoral bypass graft

AFC adult foster care
air filled cushions

AFDC Aid to Family and Dependent Children

AFE amniotic fluid embolization

AFEB afebrile

AFI amniotic fluid index

A fib atrial fibrillation

AFIP Armed Forces Institute of Pathology

AFL atrial flutter

AFLP acute fatty liver of pregnancy

AFO ankle-foot orthosis

AFP alpha-fetoprotein

AFRD acute febrile respiratory disease

AFV amniotic fluid volume

AFVSS afebrile, vital signs stable

AFX air-fluid exchange

Ag antigen

AG abdominal girth
aminoglycoside
anion gap
anti-gravity
atrial gallop

A/G albumin to globulin ratio

AGA accelerated growth area
acute gonococcal arthritis
appropriate for gestational age
average gestational age

AGD agar gel diffusion

AGE acute gastroenteritis
angle of greatest extension

AGF angle of greatest flexion

AGG	agammaglobulinemia
aggl.	agglutination
AGL	acute granulocytic leukemia
A GLAC-TO-LK	alpha galactoside leukocytes
AGN	acute glomerulonephritis
$AgNO_3$	silver nitrate
AGPT	agar-gel precipitation test
AGS	adrenogenital syndrome
AGTT	abnormal glucose tolerance test
AH	abdominal hysterectomy
	amenorrhea-hyperprolactinemia
	antihyaluronidase
A&H	accident and health (insurance)
AHA	acetohydroxamic acid
	acquired hemolytic anemia
	autoimmune hemolytic anemia
AHC	acute hemorrhagic conjunctivitis
	acute hemorrhagic cystitis
AHD	autoimmune hemolytic disease
AHE	acute hemorrhagic encephalomyelitis
AHEC	Area Health Education Center
AHF	antihemophilic factor
AHFS	American Hospital Formulary Service
AHG	antihemophilic globulin
AHGS	acute herpetic gingival stomatitis
AHL	apparent half-life
AHM	ambulatory Holter monitoring
AHN	adenomatous hyperplastic nodule
	Assistant Head Nurse
AHP	acute hemorrhagic pancreatitis
AHS	adaptive hand skills
AHT	autoantibodies to human thyroglobulin
AI	accidentally incurred
	allergy index
	aortic insufficiency
	artificial insemination
A & I	Allergy and Immunology (department)
AIA	anti-insulin antibody
	aspirin-induced asthma
AI-Ab	anti-insulin antibody
AIBF	anterior interbody fusion
AICA	anterior inferior cerebellar artery
	anterior inferior communicating artery
AICD	automatic implantable cardioverter/defibrillator
AID	acute infectious disease
	artificial insemination donor
	automatic implantable defibrillator
AIDKS	acquired immune deficiency syndrome with Kaposi's sarcoma
AIDS	acquired immune deficiency syndrome
AIE	acute inclusion body encephalitis
AIF	aortic-iliac-femoral
AIH	artificial insemination with husband's sperm
AIHA	autoimmune hemolytic anemia
AIHD	acquired immune hemolytic disease
AIIS	anterior inferior iliac spine
AILD	angioimmunoblastic lymphadenopathy (with dysproteinemia)
AIMS	Abnormal Involuntary Movement Scale
	Arthritis Impact Measurement Scales
AIN	acute interstitial nephritis
	anal intraepithelial neoplasia
AINS	anti-inflammatory non-steroidal

AION anterior ischemic optic neuropathy
AIP acute infectious polyneuritis
acute intermittent porphyria
AIR accelerated idioventricular rhythm
AIS Abbreviated Injury Score
anti-insulin serum
AIS/ISS Abbreviated Injury Scale/Injury Severity Score
AITP autoimmune thrombocytopenia purpura
AIU absolute iodine uptake
AIVR accelerated idioventricular rhythm
AJ ankle jerk
AJR abnormal jugular reflex
AK above knee (amputation)
actinic keratosis
artificial kidney
AKA above-knee amputation
alcoholic ketoacidosis
all known allergies
also known as
AL acute leukemia
argon laser
arterial line
axial length
left ear
ALA aminolevulinic acid
ALAC antibiotic-loaded acrylic cement
ALAD abnormal left axis deviation
ALARA as low as reasonably achievable
ALAT alanine transaminase (alanine aminotransferase; SGPT)
Alb albumin
ALC acute lethal catatonia
alcohol
allogeneic lymphocyte cytotoxicity
alternate level of care
alternate lifestyle checklist
ALC R alcohol rub
ALD adrenoleukodystrophy
alcoholic liver disease
aldolase
ALDOST aldosterone
ALFT abnormal liver function tests
ALG antilymphocyte globulin
ALI argon laser iridotomy
alk alkaline
ALK ISO alkaline phosphatase isoenzymes
ALK-P alkaline phosphatase
ALL acute lymphoblastic leukemia
acute lymphocytic leukemia
allergy
ALM acral lentiginous melanoma
ALMI anterolateral myocardial infarction
ALN anterior lymph node
$Al(OH)_3$ aluminum hydroxide
ALP argon laser photocoagulation
Alupent®
ALPZ alprazolam
ALS acute lateral sclerosis
advanced life support
amyotrophic lateral sclerosis
ALT alanine transaminase (SGPT)
2 alt Argon laser trabeculoplasty
every other day (this is a dangerous abbreviation)
ALTB acute laryngotracheobronchitis
ALVAD abdominal left ventricular assist device
ALWMI anterolateral wall myocardial infarct
AM adult male
amalgam
morning (a.m.)
myopic astigmatism

AMA against medical advice
American Medical Association
antimitochondrial antibody

AMAD morning admission

AMAG adrenal medullary autograft

AMAL amalgam

AMAP as much as possible

AMAT anti-malignant antibody test

A-MAT amorphous material

AMB ambulate
ambulatory
amphotericin B

AMC arm muscle circumference

AM/CR amylase to creatinine ratio

AMD age-related macular degeneration
methyldopa (alpha methyldopa)

AMegL acute megokaryoblastic leukemia

AMES-LAN American sign language

AMF autocrine motility factor

AMG acoustic myography
aminoglycoside

AMI acute myocardial infarction
amitriptyline

AML acute myelogenous leukemia

AMM agnogenic myeloid metaplasia

AMML acute myelomonocytic leukemia

AMMOL acute myelomonoblastic leukemia

AMN adrenomyeloneuropathy

amnio amniocentesis

AMN SC amniotic fluid scan

AMOL acute monoblastic leukemia

AMP adenosine monophosphate
ampicillin
ampul
amputation

A-M pr Austin-Moore prosthesis

AMPT alphamethylpara tyrosine

AMR alternating motor rates

AMS acute mountain sickness
aggravated in military service
amylase
auditory memory span

m-AMSA acridinyl anisidide

AMSIT portion of the mental status examination: A—appearance, M—mood, S—sensorium, I—intelligence, T—thought process

amt. amount

AMV assisted mechanical ventilation

AMY amylase

AN anorexia nervosa
Associate Nurse

ANA antinuclear antibody

ANAD anorexia nervosa and associated disorders

ANC absolute neutrophil count

anch anchored

ANCOVA analysis of covariance

AND anterior nasal discharge

ANDA Abbreviated New Drug Application

anes anesthesia

ANF antinuclear factor
atrial natriuretic factor

ANG angiogram

ANISO anisocytosis

ANLL acute nonlymphoblastic leukemia

ANOVA analysis of variance

ANP atrial natriuretic peptide

ANS answer
autonomic nervous system

ANT anterior
enpheptin (2-amino-5-nitrothiazol)

ante before

ANTI A:AGT anti blood group A antiglobulin test

Anti bx antibiotic

ant sag D anterior sagittal diameter

ANTU alpha naphthylthiourea

ANUG	acute necrotizing ulcerative gingivitis
ANX	anxiety
	anxious
AO	anterior oblique
	aorta
	aortic opening
	plate, screw (orthopedics)
	right ear
A & O	alert and oriented
A&O × 3	awake and oriented to person, place, and time
A&O × 4	awake and oriented to person, place, time, and date
AOAP	as often as possible
AOB	alcohol on breath
AOC	anode opening contraction
	antacid of choice
	area of concern
AOCD	anemia of chronic disease
AOD	alleged onset date
	arterial occlusive disease
	Assistant-Officer-of-the-Day
AODA	alcohol and other drug abuse
AODM	adult onset diabetes mellitus
ao-il	aorta-iliac
AOM	acute otitis media
AOO	continuous arterial asynchronous pacing
AOP	aortic pressure
AOSD	adult-onset Still's disease
AP	acute pancreatitis
	alkaline phosphatase
	angina pectoris
	antepartum
	anterior-posterior (x-ray)
	arterial pressure
	apical pulse
	appendicitis
	atrial pacing
	attending physician
	doxorubicin and cisplatin
A&P	active and present
	anterior and posterior
	assessment and plans
	auscultation and percussion
A/P	ascites/plasma ratio
$A_2 > P_2$	second aortic sound greater than second pulmonic sound
APACHE	Acute Physiology and Chronic Health Evaluation
APAP	acetaminophen
APB	abductor pollicis brevis
	atrial premature beat
APC	adenoidal-pharyngeal-conjunctival
	adenomatous polyposis of the colon and rectum
	aspirin, phenacetin, and caffeine
	atrial premature contraction
APCD	adult polycystic disease
APD	afferent pupillary defect
	aminohydroxypropylidene diphosphate
	anterior-posterior diameter
	atrial premature depolarization
	automated peritoneal dialysis
APDC	Anxiety and Panic Disorder Clinic
APE	acute psychotic episode
	acute pulmonary edema
APG	Apgar (score)
APH	adult psychiatric hospital
	alcohol-positive history
	antepartum hemorrhage
APIVR	artificial pacemaker-induced ventricular rhythm
APKD	adult polycystic kidney disease
	adult-onset polycystic kidney disease
APL	abductor pollicis longus
	accelerated painless labor
	acute promyelocytic leukemia
	anterior pituitary-like

(hormone)
chorionic gonadotropin

AP & L anteroposterior and lateral
APN acute pyelonephritis
APO doxorubicin, prednisone, and vincristine
apo E apolipoprotein E
APPG aqueous procaine penicillin G (dangerous terminology; for intramuscular use only, write as penicillin G procaine)
appr. approximate
appt. appointment
APPY appendectomy
APR abdominoperineal resection
APS Adult Psychiatric Service
APSAC anistreplase (anisoylated plasminogen streptokinase activator complex)
APSD Alzheimer's presenile dementia
aPTT activated partial thromboplastin time
APVR aortic pulmonary valve replacement
aq water
AQ accomplishment quotient
aq dest distilled water
AR active resistance
airway resistance
alcohol related
aortic regurgitation
aural rehabilitation
autorefractor
Ar argon
A&R adenoidectomy with radium
advised and released
A-R apical-radial (pulses)
ARA-A vidarabine
ARA-AC fazarabine
ARA-C cytarabine
ARB any reliable brand
ARBOR arthorpod-borne virus
ARBOW artificial rupture of bag of water
ARC anomalous retinal correspondence
AIDS related complex
American Red Cross
ARCBS American Red Cross Blood Services
ARD acute respiratory disease
adult respiratory distress
antibiotic removal device
aphakic retinal detachment
ARDS adult respiratory distress syndrome
ARE active-resistive exercises
ARF acute renal failure
acute respiratory failure
acute rheumatic fever
ARG arginine
ARI aldose reductase inhibitor
ARLD alcohol related liver disease
ARM anxiety reaction, mild
artificial rupture of membranes
ARMS amplification refractory mutation system
ARN acute retinal necrosis
AROM active range of motion
artifical rupture of membranes
ARP alcohol rehabilitation program
arr arrive
A.R.R.T. American Registry of Radiologic Technologists
ARS antirabies serum
ART Accredited Record Technician
Achilles (tendon) reflex test
acoustic reflex threshold(s)
arterial
automated reagin test (for syphilis)
ARTIC articulation
Art T art therapy
ARV AIDS related virus

ARW — Accredited Rehabilitation Worker
ARWY — airway
AS — activated sleep
anal sphincter
ankylosingspondylitis
aortic stenosis
doctor called through answering service
atropine sulfate
left ear
ASA — aspirin (acetylsalicyclic acid)
American Society of Anesthesiologists
argininosuccinate
ASA I — Healthy patient with localized pathological process
ASA II — A patient with mild to moderate systemic disease
ASA III — A patient with severe systemic disease limiting activity but not incapacitating
ASA IV — A patient with incapacitating systemic disease
ASA V — Moribund patient not expected to live.
(These are American Society of Anesthesiologists' patient classifications. Emergency operations are designated by "E" after the classification).
ASAA — acquired severe aplastic anemia
ASACL — American Society of Anesthesiologists Classification
AS/AI — aortic stenosis/aortic insufficiency
ASAP — as soon as possible
ASAT — aspartate transaminase (aspartate aminotransferase) (SGOT)
ASB — anesthesia standby
asymptomatic bacteriuria
ASC — altered state of consciousness
ambulatory surgery center
anterior subcapsular cataract
antimony sulfur colloid
ascorbic acid
ASCVD — arteriosclerotic cardiovascular disease
ASD — atrial septal defect
ASDH — acute subdural hematoma
ASE — acute stress erosion
ASH — asymmetric septal hypertrophy
AsH — hypermetropic astigmatism
ASHD — arteriosclerotic heart disease
ASI — Anxiety Status Inventory
ASIS — anterior superior iliac spine
ASK — antistreptokinase
ASL — antistreptolysin (titer)
ASLO — antistreptolysin-O
AsM — myopic astigmatism
ASMA — anti-smooth muscle antibody
ASMI — anteroseptal myocardial infarction
ASO — aldicarb sulfoxide
antistreptolysin-O titer
arteriosclerosis obliterans
automatic stop order
ASOT — antistreptolysin-O titer
ASP — acute suppurative parotitis
acute symmetric polyarthritis
aspartic acid
ASPVD — arteriosclerotic peripheral vascular disease
ASS — anterior superior supine
assessment
asst — assistant
AST — aspartate transaminase (SGOT)
astemizole
astigmatism
AS TOL — as tolerated
ASTIG — astigmatism

ASTZ	antistreptozyme test
ASU	acute stroke unit ambulatory surgical unit
ASV	antisnake venom
ASVD	arteriosclerotic vessel disease
ASYM	asymmetric (al)
AT	activity therapy (therapist) antithrombin applanation tonometry atraumatic
AT 10	dihydrotachysterol
ATB	antibiotic
ATC	alcoholism therapy classes around the clock
ATD	antithyroid drug(s) autoimmune thyroid disease
At Fib	atrial fibrillation
AT III FUN	antithrombin III functional
ATG	antithymocyte globulin
ATHR	angina threshold heart rate
ATL	Achilles tendon lengthening adult T-cell leukemia anterior tricuspid leaflet atypical lymphocytes
ATLS	advanced trauma life support
ATM	acute transverse myelitis
At ma	atrial milliamp atmosphere
ATN	acute tubular necrosis
ATNC	atraumatic normocephalic
aTNM	autopsy staging of cancer
ATNR	asymmetrical tonic neck reflux
ATP	addiction treatment program adenosine triphosphate
ATPase	adenosine triphosphatase
ATPS	ambient temperature & pressure, saturated with water vapor
ATR	Achilles tendon reflex atrial
atr fib	atrial fibrillation
ATRO	atropine
ATS	antitetanic serum (tetanus antitoxin) anxiety tension state
ATSO4	atropine sulfate
ATT	arginine tolerance test
at. wt	atomic weight
AU	allergenic units both ears
Au	gold
198_{Au}	radioactive gold
AUB	abnormal uterine bleeding
AUC	area under the curve
AUD COMP	auditory comprehension
AUGIB	acute upper gastrointestinal bleeding
AUL	acute undifferentiated leukemia
AUR	acute urinary retention
AUS	acute urethral syndrome auscultation
AV	arteriovenous atrioventricular auditory visual
AVA	aortic valve atresia arteriovenous anastomosis
AVD	aortic valve disease apparent volume of distribution
AVDP	asparaginase, vincristine daunorubicin, and prednisone avoirdupois
$AVDO_2$	arteriovenous oxygen difference
AVF	arteriovenous fistula augmented unipolar foot (left leg)
avg	average
AVGs	ambulatory visit groups
AVH	acute viral hepatitis
AVJR	atrioventricular junctional rhythm
AVL	augmented unipolar left (left arm)
AVM	atriovenous malformation
AVN	arteriovenous nicking atrioventricular node avascular necrosis

AVNRT	AV nodal reentry tachycardia
AVOC	avocation
AVP	arginine vasopressin
AVR	aortic valve replacement
	augmented unipolar right (right arm)
AVS	atriovenous shunt
AVSS	afebrile, vital signs stable
AVT	atrioventricular tachycardia
	atypical ventricular tachycardia
AW	abdominal wall
	abnormal wave
A/W	able to work
A&W	alive and well
AWA	as well as
A waves	atrial contraction waves
AWDW	assault with a deadly weapon
AWI	anterior wall infarct
AWMI	anterior wall myocardial infarction
AWO	airway obstruction
AWOL	absent without leave
ax	axillary
AXR	abdomen x-ray
AXT	alternating exotropia
AZA	azathioprine
5 AZA	azacitidine
AZQ	diaziquone
AZT	zidovudine (azidothymidine)
A-Z test	Ascheim-Zondek test diagnostic test for pregnancy

B

B	bacillus
	bands
B	bilateral
	black
	bloody
	both
	buccal
B_1	thiamine HCl
B_2	riboflavin
B_6	pyridoxine HCl
B_7	biotin
B_8	adenosine phosphate
B_{12}	cyanocobalamin
Ba	barium
BA	backache
	benzyl alcohol
	bile acid
	blood alcohol
	bone age
	Bourns assist
	branchial artery
	bronchial asthma
B > A	bone greater than air
B & A	brisk and active
B&B	bowel and bladder
Bab	Babinski
BAC	benzalkonium chloride
	blood alcohol concentration
	buccoaxiocervical
BACON	bleomycin, doxorubicin, lomustine, vincristine, and mechlorethamine
BACOP	bleomycin, adriamycin, cyclophosphamide, vincristine, and prednisone
BACT	bacteria
BAD	dipolar affective disorder
BaE	barium enema
BAE	bronchial artery embolization
BAEP	brain stem auditory evoked potential
BAERs	brain stem auditory evoked responses
BAL	balance
	blood alcohol level
	British antilewisite (dimercaprol)
	bronchoalveolar lavage
BALB	binaural alternate loudness balance
BaM	barium meal
BAND	band neutrophil (stab)
BANS	back, arm, neck and scalp
BAO	basal acid output
BAP	blood agar plate

Barb	barbiturate
BARN	bilateral acute retinal necrosis
BAS	boric acid solution
BaS	barium swallow
BASK	basket cells
baso.	basophil
BASO STIP	basophilic stippling
batt	battery
BAVP	balloon aortic valvuloplasty
BAW	bronchoalveolar washing
BB	baby boy
	backboard
	bad breath
	bed bath
	bed board
	beta blocker
	blanket bath
	blood bank
	blow bottle
	blue bloaters
	body belts
	both bones
	bowel or bladder
	breakthrough bleeding
	breast biopsy
	buffer base
B/B	backward bending
BBA	born before arrival
BBB	blood-brain barrier
	bundle branch block
BBBB	bilateral bundle branch block
BBD	before bronchodilator
	benign breast disease
BBM	banked breast milk
BBS	bilateral breath sounds
BBT	basal body temperature
BB to MM	belly button to medial malleolus
B Bx	breast biopsy
BC	back care
	bed and chair
	birth control
	blood culture
	Blue Cross
	bone conduction
	Bourn control
B/C	because
	blood urea nitrogen/creatinine ratio
B&C	bed and chair
	biopsy and curettage
	board and care
	breathed and cried
BC/BS	Blue Cross/Blue Shield
BCA	balloon catheter angioplasty
	basal cell atypia
	brachiocephalic artery
BCAA	branched-chain amino acids
B. cat	Branhamella catarrhalis
B-CAVe	bleomycin, lomustine, doxorubicin, and vinblastine
BCC	basal cell carcinoma
	birth control clinic
BCCa	basal cell carcinoma
BCD	basal cell dysplasia
BCE	basal cell epithelioma
B cell	large lymphocyte
BCG	bacillus Calmette-Guérin vaccine
	bicolor guaiac
BCL	basic cycle length
BCM	birth control medication
BCNP	Board Certified Nuclear Pharmacist
BCNU	carmustine
BCP	birth control pills
	carmustine, cyclophosphamide, and prednisone
BCS	battered child syndrome
	Budd-Chiari syndrome
BCU	burn care unit
BD	band neutrophil
	base down
	bile duct
	birth date
	birth defect
	blood donor
	brain dead
	bronchial drainage
BDAE	Boston Diagnostic Aphasia Examination

BDBS	Bonnet-Dechaume-Blanc Syndrome
BDC	burn-dressing change
BDE	bile duct exploration
BDF	black divorced female
BDI SF	Beck's Depression Index-Short Form
BDL	below detectable limits
	bile duct ligation
BDM	black divorced male
B-DOPA	bleomycin, dacarbazine, vincristine, prednisone, and doxorubicin
BDP	beclomethasone diproprionate
BDR	background diabetic retinopathy
BE	bacterial endocarditis
	barium enema
	base excess
	below elbow
	bread equivalent
	breast examination
B↑E	both upper extremities
B E	both lower extremities
B & E	brisk and equal
BEA	below elbow amputation
BEAM	brain electrical activity mapping
BEC	bacterial endocarditis
BEE	basal energy expenditure
BEF	bronchoesophageal fistula
Beh Sp	behavior specialist
BEI	butanol-extractable iodine
BEP	bleomycin, etoposide, and cisplatin
	brain stem evoked potentials
BEV	billion electron volts
	bleeding esophageal varices
BF	black female
	boyfriend
	breakfast fed
	breast-feed
BFA	baby for adoption
	bifemoral arteriogram
BFC	benign febrile convulsion
BFL	breast firm and lactating
BFM	black married female
BFP	biologic false positive
B. frag	*Bacillus fragilis*
BFT	bentonite flocculation test
	biofeedback training
BFU_e	erythroid burst-forming unit
BG	baby girl
	blood glucose
	bone graft
B-G	Bender-Gestalt (test)
B-GA-LACTO	beta galactosidase
BGC	basal-ganglion calcification
BGDC	Bartholin gland duct cyst
BGL	blood glucose level
BH	breath holding
BHC	benzene hexachloride
BHD	carmustine, hydroxyurea, and dacarbazine
B-HEXOS-A-LK	beta hexosaminidase A leukocytes
BHI	biosynthetic human insulin
BHN	bridging hepatic necrosis
BHS	beta-hemolytic streptococci
	breath-holding spell
BHT	breath hydrogen test
BI	base in
	brain injury
	bowel impaction
BIB	brought in by
BIC	brain injury center
Bicarb	bicarbonate
BICROS	bilateral contralateral routing of signals
BID	brought in dead
	twice daily
BIF	bifocal
BIG 6	analysis of 6 serum components (see SMA 6)
BIH	benign intracranial hypertension
	bilateral inguinal hernia
BIL	bilateral
	brother-in-law
BILAT SLC	bilateral short leg case

BILAT SXO	bilateral salpingo-oophorectomy
Bili	bilirubin
BILI-C	conjugated bilirubin
BIMA	bilateral internal mammary arteries
BIN	twice a night (this is a dangerous abbreviation)
BIOF	biofeedback
BiPD	biparietal diameter
bisp	bispinous diameter
B.I.W.	twice a week (this is a dangerous abbreviation)
BIZ-PLT	bizarre platelets
BJ	Bence-Jones
	biceps jerk
	bone and joint
BJE	bone and joint examination
BJM	bones, joints, and muscles
BJP	Bence-Jones protein
BK	below knee (amputation)
	bradykinin
	bullous keratopathy
BKA	below knee amputation
BKC	blepharokerato-conjunctivitis
bkft	breakfast
Bkg	background
BKU	base up
BKWP	below-knee walking plaster (cast)
BL	baseline (fetal heart rate)
	bland
	blast cells
	blood level
	blood loss
	bronchial lavage
	Burkitt's lymphoma
BLB	Boothby-Lovelace-Bulbulian (oxygen mask)
BLBK	blood bank
BL = BS	bilateral equal breath sounds
bl cult	blood culture
bldg	bleeding
bld tm	bleeding time
BLE	both lower extremities
BLEO	bleomycin sulfate
BLESS	bath, laxative, enema, shampoo, and shower
BLL	bilateral lower lobe
BLM	bleomycin sulfate
BLOBS	bladder obstruction
BLPO	beta-lactamase-producing organism
BLQ	both lower quadrants
BLR	blood flow rate
BLS	basic life support
B.L. unit	Bessey-Lowry units
BM	black male
	bone marrow
	bowel movement
	breast milk
BMA	bone marrow aspirate
BMC	bone marrow cells
BMD	Becker muscular dystrophy
	bone marrow depression
	bone mineral density
BME	brief maximal effort
BMI	body mass index
BMJ	bones, muscles, joints
BMK	birthmark
BMM	black married male
BMP	behavior management plan
BMR	basal metabolic rate
	best motor response
BMT	bilateral myringotomy and tubes
	bone marrow transplant
BMTT	bilateral myringotomy with tympanic tubes
BMTU	bone marrow transplant unit
BNC	bladder neck contracture
BNCT	boron neutron capture therapy
BNO	bladder neck obstruction
BNR	bladder neck retraction
BO	behavior objective
	body odor
	bowel obstruction
B & O	belladonna & opium (suppositories)
BOA	born on arrival
	born out of asepsis
BOB	ball on back

BOD	bilateral orbital decompression
Bod Units	Bodansky units
BOE	bilateral otitis externa
BOLD	bleomycin, vincristine, (Oncovin) lomustine, and dacarbazine
BOM	bilateral otitis media
BOMA	bilateral otitis media, acute
BOO	bladder outlet obstruction
BOOP	bronchitis obliterans with organized pneumonia
BOT	base of tongue
BOW	bag of water
BP	bathroom privileges
	bed pan
	benzoyl peroxide
	bipolar
	birthplace
	blood pressure
	bypass
	British Pharmacopeia
BPI	bipolar affective disorder, Type I
BPD	biparietal diameter
	borderline personality disorder
	bronchopulmonary dysplasia
BPd	diastolic blood pressure
BPF	bronchopleural fistula
BPH	benign prostatic hypertrophy
BPG	bypass graft
BPL	benzylpenicilloylpoly-lysine
BPLA	blood pressure, left arm
BPM	beats per minute
	breaths per minute
BPN	bacitracin, polymyxin B, and neomycin sulfate
BPPP	bilateral pedal pulses present
BPR	blood per rectum
	blood pressure recorder
BPRS	Brief Psychiatric Rating Scale
BPS	bilateral partial salpingectomy
BPs	systolic blood pressure
BPSD	bronchopulmonary segmental drainage
BPV	benign paroxysmal vertigo
	bovine papilloma virus
Bq	becquerel
BR	bathroom
	bedrest
	Benzing retrograde
	blink reflex
	bowel rest
	bridge
	brown
Br	bromide
BRA	brain
BRADY	bradycardia
BRAO	branch retinal artery occlusion
BRAT	bananas, rice cereal, applesauce, and toast
BRATT	bananas, rice, cereal, applesauce, tea, & toast
BRB	blood-retinal barrier
	bright red blood
BRBR	bright red blood per rectum
BRBPR	bright red blood per rectum
BRCM	below right costal margin
BRJ	brachial radialis jerk
BRM	biological response modifiers
BRO	brother
BRP	bathroom privileges
BR RAO	branch retinal artery occlusion
BR RVO	branch retinal vein occlusion
BRVO	branch retinal vein occlusion
BS	bedside
	before sleep
	Bennett seal
	blood sugar
	Blue Shield
	bowel sounds
	breath sounds

B & S	Bartholin & Skene (glands)
BSA	body surface area
	bowel sounds active
BSAB	Balthazar Scales of Adaptive Behavior
BSB	bedside bag
	body surface burned
BSC	bedside care
	bedside commode
	burn scar contracture
BSD	baby soft diet
	bedside drainage
BSE	breast self-examination
BSepF	black separated female
BSepM	black separated male
BSER	brain stem evoked responses
BSF	black single female
	busulfan
BSGA	beta Streptococcus group A
BSI	body substance isolation
	brainstem injury
BSL	blood sugar level
BSM	black single male
BSN	Bachelor of Science in Nursing
BS L base	breath sounds diminished, left base
BSN	bowel sounds normal
BSNA	bowel sounds normal and active
BSNT	breast soft and nontender
BSO	bilateral salpingo-oophorectomy
BSOM	bilateral serous otitis media
BSP	bromsulphalein
BSPA	bowel sounds present and active
BSPM	body surface potential mapping
BSS	bedside scale
	bismuth subsalicylate
BSS®	balanced salt solution
	black silk sutures
BSSG	sitogluside
BSSS	benign sporadic sleep spikes
BST	bedside testing
	brief stimulus therapy
BSU	Bartholin, Skene's, urethra
BSW	Bachelor of Social Work
BT	bedtime
	bleeding time
	bituberous
	bladder tumor
	blood type
	blood transfusion
	brain tumor
	breast tumor
BTB	break-through bleeding
BTBV	beat to beat variability
BTC	bladder tumor check
	by the clock
BTE	behind-the-ear (hearing aid)
BTF	blenderized tube feeding
BTFS	breast tumor frozen section
BTG	beta thromboglobulin
BTL	bilateral tubal ligation
BTPS	body temperature pressure saturated
BTR	bladder tumor recheck
BU	below umbilicus
	Bodansky units
	burn unit
BUdR	bromodeoxyurdine
BUE	both upper extremities
BUFA	baby up for adoption
BUN	blood urea nitrogen
	bunion
BUR	back-up rate (ventilator)
Burd	Burdick suction
BUS	Bartholin, urethral, and Skene's glands
BV	bacterial vaginitis
	biological value
	blood volume
BVAD	bi-ventricular assist device
BVE	blood volume expander
BVL	bilateral vas ligation
BVO	branch vein occlusion
BVRT	Benton Visual Retention Test
BW	birth weight

	bite-wing (radiograph)
	body water
	body weight
B & W	Black and White (milk of magnesia & aromatic cascara fluidextract)
BWA	bed wetter admission
BWCS	bagged white cell study
BWFI	bacteriostatic water for injection
BWidF	black widowed female
BWidM	black widowed male
BWS	battered woman syndrome
ΦBZ	phenylbutazone
Bx	biopsy
BX BS	Blue Cross and Blue Shield
BXM	B cell crossmatch
BZDZ	benzodiazepine

C

C	ascorbic acid
	carbohydrate
	Catholic
	Caucasian
	Celsius
	centigrade
	clubbing
	cyanosis
	hundred
c̄	with
$C_1 \ldots C_7$	cervical nerve 1 through 7
	cervical vertebra 1 through 7
C_1 to C_9	precursor molecules of the complement system
CII	controlled substance, class 2
C_{II}	second cranial nerve
CA	carcinoma
	cardiac arrest
	carotid artery
	celiac artery
	chronologic age
	Cocaine Anonymous
	compressed air
	coronary angioplasty
	coronary artery
Ca	calcium
C&A	Clinitest® and Acetest®
CAA	crystalline amino acids
CAB	catheter-associated bacteriuria
	coronary artery bypass
CABG	coronary artery bypass graft
CaBI	calcium bone index
CABS	coronary artery bypass surgery
CACI	computer assisted continuous infusion
$CaCO_3$	calcium carbonate
CACP	cisplatin
CAD	coronary artery disease
CAE	cellulose acetate electrophoresis
	cyclophosphamide, doxorubicin, and etoposide
CAEC	cardiac arrhythmia evaluation center
CaEDTA	calcium disodium edetate
CAF	cyclophosphamide, doxorubicin, and fluorouracil
CAFT	Clinitron air fluidized therapy
CAG	continuous ambulatory gamma globin (infusion)
CaG	calcium gluconate
CAH	chronic active hepatitis
	chronic aggressive hepatitis
	congenital adrenal hyperplasia
CAL	callus
	calories (cal)
	chronic airflow limitation
cal ct	calorie count
CALD	chronic active liver disease
CALGB	Cancer and Leukemia Group B
CALLA	common acute lymphoblastic leukemia antigen
CAM	Caucasian adult male
CAMF	cyclophosphamide,

adriamycin, methotrexate, and fluorouracil
CAMP cyclophosphamide, doxorubicin, methotrexate, and procarbazine
CAN cord around neck
CA/N child abuse and neglect
CANC cancelled
CAO chronic airway (airflow) obstruction
CAP capsule
chloramphenicol
community-acquired pneumonia
compound action potentials
cyclophosphamide, doxorubicin, and cisplatin
CaP carcinoma of the prostate
Ca/P calcium to phosphorus ratio
CAPB central auditory processing battery
CAPD chronic ambulatory peritoneal dialysis
CAR cardiac ambulation routine
CARB carbohydrate
CAS carotid artery stenosis
CASHD coronary arteriosclerotic heart disease
CASP Child Analytic Study Program
CASS computer aided sleep system
CAT cataract
children's apperception test
computed axial tomography
cath. catheter
catheterization
CAV computer-aided ventilation
cyclophosphamide, doxorubicin, and vincristine
CAVB complete atrioventricular block
CAVC common arterioventricular canal
CAVH continuous ateriovenous hemofiltration
CAV-P-VP cyclophosphamide, doxorubicin, vincristine, cisplatin, and etoposide
CB cesarean birth
chair and bed
chronic bronchitis
code blue
C & B chair and bed
crown and bridge
CBA chronic bronchitis and asthma
CBC carbenicillin
complete blood count
CBD closed bladder drainage
common bile duct
CBDE common bile duct exploration
CBF cerebral blood blow
CBFS cerebral blood flow studies
CBFV cerebral blood flow velocity
CBG capillary blood glucose
CBI continuous bladder irrigation
CBN chronic benign neutropenia
CBP chronic benign pain
CBPS coronary bypass surgery
CBR carotid bodies resected
chronic bedrest
complete bedrest
CBRAM controlled partial rebreathing-anesthesia method
CBS chronic brain syndrome
Cruveilhier-Baumgarten syndrome
CBZ carbamazepine
CC cardiac catheterization
cerebral concussion
chief complaint
chronic complainer

circulatory collapse
clean catch (urine)
coracoclavicular
cord compression
corpus collosum
creatinine clearance
critical condition
cubic centimeter (cc), (mL)
with correction (with glasses)

C/C — cholecystectomy and operative cholangiogram
complete upper and lower dentures

C & C — cold and clammy

CCA — circumflex coronary artery
common carotid artery
concentrated care area

CCAP — capsule cartilage articular preservation

CCB — calcium channel blocker(s)

CCC — Cancer Care Center
child care clinic
Comprehensive Cancer Center

CC & C — colony count and culture

CCC-A — Certificate of Clinical Competence in Audiology

CCC-SP — Certificate of Clinical Competence in Speech-Language Pathology

CCD — childhood celiac disease

CCE — clubbing, cyanosis, and edema
countercurrent electrophoresis

CCF — compound comminuted fracture
crystal-induced chemotactic factor

CCFE — cyclophosphamide, cisplatin, fluorouracil, and estramustine

CCHD — cyanotic congenital heart disease

CCI — chronic coronary insufficiency

CCK — cholecystokinin

CCK-OP — cholecystokinin octapeptide

CCK-PZ — cholecystokininpancreozymin

CCL — cardiac catheterization laboratory
critical condition list

CCl_4 — carbon tetrachloride

CCM — cyclophosphamide, lomustine, and methotrexate

CCMSU — clean catch midstream urine

CCMU — critical care medicine unit

CCNU — lomustine

C-collar — cervical collar

CCPD — continuous cycling (cyclical) peritoneal dialysis

CCR — cardiac catheterization recovery
continuous complete remission

C_{cr} — creatinine clearance

CCRC — continuing care residential community

CCRN — Certified Critical Care Registered Nurse

CCRU — critical care recovery unit

CCT — calcitriol
closed cerebral trauma
congenitally corrected transposition (of the great vessels)
crude coal tar

CCTGA — congenitally corrected transposition of the great arteries

CCT in PET — crude coal tar in petroleum

CCTV — closed circuit television

CCU — coronary care unit
critical care unit

CCUA — clean catch urinalysis

CCUP — colpocystourethropexy

CCW childcare worker
counterclockwise
CCX complications
CD cadaver donor
cesarean delivery
childhood disease
character disorder
common duct
communication disorders
complicated delivery
continuous drainage
convulsive disorder
Crohn's Disease
cytarabine and daunorubicin
C/D cigarettes per day
cup to disc ratio
C&D curettage and desiccation
cytoscopy and dilatation
CDA chenodeoxycholic acid (chenodiol)
congenital dyserythropoietic anemia
CDAI Crohn's Disease Activity Index
CDAK Cordis Dow Artificial Kidney
CDB cough, and deep breath
CDC calculated day of confinement
cancer detection center
carboplatin, doxorubicin, and cyclophosphamide
Centers for Disease Control
chenodeoxycholic acid
CDCA chenodeoxycholic acid (chenodiol)
CDD Certificate of Disability for Discharge
CDDP cisplatin
CDE canine distemper encephalitis
Certified Diabetes Educator
common duct exploration
CDH chronic daily headache
congenital diaphragmatic hernia
congenital dislocation of hip
congenital dysplasia of the hip
CDK climatic droplet keratopathy
CDLE chronic discoid lupus erythematosus
CDP Child Development Program
CDQ corrected development quotient
CDR continuing disability review
CDR(H) cup-to-disc ratio horizontal
CDR(V) cup-to-disc ratio vertical
CDU chemical dependency unit
CDV canine distemper virus
CDX chlordiazepoxide
cdyn dynamic compliance
CE California encephalitis
cardiac enlargement
cardioesophageal
cataract extraction
central episiotomy
community education
continuing education
contrast echocardiology
C&E consultation and examination
cough and exercise
curettage and electrodesiccation
CEA carcinoembryonic antigen
carotid endarterectomy
CEC Council for Exceptional Children
CECT contrast enhancement computed tomography
CEI continuous extravascular infusion
CEL cardiac exercise laboratory
CEO chief executive officer
CEP cognitive evoked potential
congenital erythropoietic porphyria
countercurrent electrophoresis

CEPH cephalic
cephalosporin
CEPH FLOC cephalin flocculation
CER conditioned emotional response
CE&R central episiotomy & repair
CERA cortical evoked response audiometry
CERD chronic end-stage renal disease
CERULO ceruloplasmin
CERV cervical
CES cognitive environmental stimulation
CEV cyclophosphamide, etoposide, and vincristine
CF calcium leucovorin (citrovorum factor)
cancer-free
cardiac failure
Caucasian female
cephalothin
Christmas factor
cisplatin and fluorouracil
complement fixation
contractile force
count fingers
cystic fibrosis
CFA common femoral artery
complete Freund's adjuvant
CFAC complement-fixing antibody consumption
C-factor cleverness factor
CFF critical fusion (flicker) frequency
CFL cisplatin, fluorouracil, and leucovorin calcium
CFM close fitting mask
cyclophosphamide, fluorouracil, and citoxantrone
CFNS chills, fever, and night sweats
CFP cystic fibrosis protein
CFPT cyclophosphamide, fluorouracil, prednisone, and tamoxifen
CFS cancer family syndrome
Child and Family Service
chronic fatigue syndrome
CFT complement fixation test
CF test complement fixation test
CFU colony forming units
CFU-S colony forming unit—spleen
CG cholecystogram
contact guarding
CGB chronic gastrointestinal (tract) bleeding
CGD chronic granulomatous disease
CGI Clinical Global Impressions (scale)
CGL chronic granulocytic leukemia
with correction/with glasses
CGN chronic glomerulonephritis
CGTT cortisol glucose tolerance test
CH chest
chief
child (children)
chronic
cluster headache
congenital hypothyroidism
convalescent hospital
crown-heal
c̄ hold withhold
ch[1] Christ Church
chromosone
CHAD cyclophosphamide, adriamycin, cisplatin, and hexamethylmelamine
CHAI continuous hepatic artery infusion
CHAM-OCA cyclophosphamide, hydroxyurea, dactinomycin, methotrexate, vincristine, leucovorin, and doxorubicin
CHAP child health associate

	practitioner
	cyclophosphamide, hexamethylmelamine, doxorubicin, and cisplatin
CHB	complete heart block
CH_3–CCNU	semustine
CHD	center hemodialysis
	childhood diseases
	chronic hemodialysis
	common hepatic duct
	congenital heart disease
	coordinate home care
ChemoRx	chemotherapy
CHF	congestive heart failure
	Crimean hemorrhagic fever
CHFV	combined high frequency of ventilation
CHG	change
CHI	closed head injury
	creatinine-height index
CHIP	iproplatin
Chix	chickenpox
CHO	carbohydrate
chol	cholesterol
CHOP	cyclophosphamide, doxorubicin, vincristine, prednisone
CHPX	chickenpox
chr.	chronic
CHRS	congenital hereditary retinoschisis
CHS	Chediak-Higashi syndrome
CHU	closed head unit
CI	cardiac index
	cesium implant
	cochlear implant
	complete iridectomy
	coronary insufficiency
Ci	curie(s)
CIA	chronic idiopathic anhidrosis
CIAA	competitive insulin autoantibodies
CIAED	collagen induced autoimmune ear disease
CIB	Carnation Instant Breakfast
	crying-induced bronchospasm
	cytomegalic inclusion bodies
CIBD	chronic inflammatory bowel disease
CIBP	chronic intractable benign pain
CIC	circulating immune complexes
	coronary intensive care
CICE	combined intracapsular cataract extraction
CICU	cardiac intensive care unit
CID	cervical immobilization device
	cytomegalic inclusion disease
CIDP	chronic inflammatory demyelinating polyradineuropathy
CIDS	cellular immunodeficiency syndrome
	continuous insulin delivery system
CIE	counterimmunoelectro-phoresis
	crossed immunoelectro-phoresis
CIEA	continuous infusion epidural analgesia
CIEP	counterimmunoelectro-phoresis
CIG	cigarettes
CIHD	chronic ischemic heart disease
CIIA	common internal iliac artery
CIN	cervical intraepithelial neoplasia
	chronic interstitial nephritis
CINE	chemotherapy-induced nausea and emesis
	cineangiogram
CIP	Cardiac Injury Panel
CIPD	chronic intermittent peritoneal dialysis
Circ	circulation

	circumcision
	circumference
circ. & sen.	circulation and sensation
CIS	carcinoma in situ
CISCA	cisplatin, cyclophosphamide, and doxorubicin
Cis-DDP	cisplatin
CIT	conventional immunosuppressive therapy
	conventional insulin therapy
CIU	chronic idiopathic urticaria
CJD	Creutzfeldt-Jakob Disease
CK	check
	creatine kinase
CK-BB	creatine kinase BB band
CKC	cold knife conization
CK-ISO	creatine kinase isoenzyme
CK-MB	creatine kinase MB band
CK MM	creatine kinase MM band
CKW	clockwise
Cl	chloride
CL	clear liquid
	cleft lip
	cloudy
	critical list
	lung compliance
C_L	compliance of the lungs
CLA	community living arrangements
Clav	clavicle
CLB	chlorambucil
CLBBB	complete left bundle branch block
CLC	cork leather and celastic (orthotic)
CL/CP	cleft lip and cleft palate
CLD	chronic liver disease
	chronic lung disease
CLE	continuous lumbar epidural (anesthetic)
CLF	cholesterol-lecithin flocculation
CLH	chronic lobular hepatitis
CLL	chronic lymphocytic leukemia
CLLE	columnar-lined lower esophagus
cl liq	clear liquid
CLO	close
	cod liver oil
CL & P	cleft lip & palate
CLRO	community leave for reorientation
CLT	chronic lymphocytic thyroiditis
CL VOID	clean voided specimen
clysis	hypodermoclysis
cm	centimeter
CM	capreomycin
	cardiac monitor
	Caucasian male
	centimeter (cm)
	chondromalacia
	cochlear microphonics
	common migraine
	continuous murmur
	contrast media
	costal margin
	cow's milk
	culture media
	cystic mesothelioma
	tomorrow morning (this is a danger abbreviation)
cm^3	cubic centimeter
CMA	compound myopic astigmatism
CMAF	centrifuged microaggregate filter
CMBBT	cervical mucous basal body temperature
CMC	carpal metacarpal (joint)
	carboxymethylcellulose
	chloramphenicol
	chronic mucocutaneous candidosis
CMD	cytomegalic disease
CME	cervicomediastinal exploration (examination)
	continuing medical education
	cystoid macular edema
CMER	current medical evidence of record

CMF cyclophosphamide, methotrexate and fluorouracil

CMFP cyclophosphamide, methotrexate, fluorouracil, and prednisone

CMFVP cyclophosphamide, methotrexate, fluorouracil, vincristine, and prednisone

CMG cystometrogram

CMGN chronic membranous glomerulonephritis

CMHC community mental health center

CMHN Community Mental Health Nurse

CMI cell-mediated immunity
Cornell Medical Index

CMIR cell mediated immune response

CMJ carpometacarpal joint

CMK congenital multicystic kidney

CML cell-mediated lympholysis
chronic myelogenous leukemia

CMM cutaneous malignant melanoma

CMML chronic myelomacrocytic leukemia

CMO Chief Medical Officer

CMP cardiomyopathy
chondromalacia patellae

CMR cerebral metabolic rate

CMRNG chromosomally mediated resistant *Neisseria gonorrhoeae*

$CMRO_2$ cerebral metabolic rate for oxygen

CMS circulation motion sensation

CMSUA clean midstream urinalysis

CMT cutis marmorata telangiectasia

CMV cisplatin, methotrexate, and vinblastine
controlled mechanical ventilation
cool mist vaporizer
cytomegalovirus

CN cranial nerve
tomorrow night (this is a dangerous abbreviation)

Cn cyanide

C/N contrast-to-noise ratio

CN II–XII cranial nerves 2–12

CNA chart not available

CNAG chronic narrow angle glaucoma

CNCbl cyanocobalamin

CND canned
cannot determine

CNDC chronic nonspecific diarrhea of childhood

CNE chronic nervous exhaustion

CNF cyclophosphamide, mitoxantrone, and fluorouracil

CNH central neurogenic hypernea

CNM certified nurse midwife

CNN congenital nevocytic nevus

CNOR Certified Nurse, Operating Room

CNRN Certified Neurosurgical Registered Nurse

CNS central nervous system
Clinical Nurse Specialist

CNT could not test

CO carbon monoxide
cardiac output
castor oil
centric occlusion
cervical orthosis
court order

Co cobalt

C/O check out
complained of
complaints
under care of

CO_2 carbon dioxide

CoA coarctation of the aorta

COAD	chronic obstructive airway disease
	chronic obstructive arterial disease
COAG	chronic open angle glaucoma
COAGSC	coagulation screen
COAP	cyclophosphamide, vincristine, cytarabine, and prednisone
COB	cisplatin, vincristine, and bleomycin
COBS	chronic organic brain syndrome
COBT	chronic obstruction of biliary tract
COCCIO	coccideimycosis
COD	cause of death
	codeine
	condition on discharge
COD-MD	cerebro-ocular-dysplasia-muscular dystrophy
CODO	codocytes
COEPS	cortically originating extrapyramidal symptoms
COG	Central Oncology Group
	cognitive function tests
COGN	cognition
COH	carbohydrate
COHB	carboxyhemoglobin
Coke	Coca-Cola®
	cocaine
COLD	chronic obstructive lung disease
COLD A	cold agglutin titer
Collyr	eye wash
col/ml	colonies per milliliter
colp	colporrhaphy
COM	chronic otitis media
COMF	comfortable
COMLA	cyclophosphamide, vincristine, methotrexate, calcium leucovorin, and cytarabine
COMP	complications
	compound
	compress
	cyclophosphamide, vincristine, methotrexate, and prednisone
COMT	catechol-o-methyl transferase
CON A	concanavalin A
conc.	concentrated
CONG	congenital
	gallon
CONPA-DRI I	cyclophosphamide, vincristine, doxorubicin, and melphalan
CONPA-DRI II	conpadri I plus high-dose methotrexate
CONPA-DRI III	conpadri I plus intensified doxorubicin
cont	continuous
	contusions
CONTU	contusion
COP	cicatricial ocular pemphigoid
	colloid osmotic pressure
	cycophosphamide, vincristine, and prednisone
COPD	chronic obstructive pulmonary disease
COPE	chronic obstructive pulmonary emphysema
COPP	cyclophosphamide, vincristine, procarbazine, and prednisone
cor	coronary
CORT	Certified Operating Room Technician
COS	clinically observed seizure
COT	content of thought
COTA	Certified Occupational Therapy Assistant
COTX	cast off to x-ray
COU	cardiac observation unit
COX	Coxsackie virus
CP	centric position
	cerebral palsy
	Certified Paramedic
	chest pain

chloroquine-primaquine combination tablets
chondromalacia patella
chronic pain
cleft palate
convenience package
creatine phosphokinase
cyclophosphamide and cisplatin

C&P complete and pushing
cystoscopy and pyelography

CPA cardiopulmonary arrest
carotid photoangiography
cerebellar pontile angle
conditioned play audiometry
costophrenic angle
cyclophosphamide

CPAF chlorpropamide-alcohol flush

CPAP continuous positive airway pressure

CPB cardiopulmonary bypass
competitive protein binding

CPBA competitive protein-binding assay

CPC cerebral palsy clinic
chronic passive congestion
clinicopathologic conference

CPCR cardiopulmonary-cerebral resuscitation

CPCS clinical pharmacokinctics consulting service

CPD cephalopelvic disproportion
chorioretinopathy and pituitary dysfunction
chronic peritoneal dialysis
citrate-phosphate-dextrose

CPDA-1 citrate-phosphate-dextrose-adenine

CPDD calcium pyrophosphate deposition disease

CPE cardiogenic pulmonary edema
chronic pulmonary emphysema
complete physical examination

CPGN chronic progressive glomerulonephritis

CPH chronic persistent hepatitis

CPI constitutionally psychopathia inferior

CPID chronic pelvic inflammatory disease

CPIP chronic pulmonary insufficiency of prematurity

CPK creatinine phosphokinase (BB, MB, MM are isoenzymes)

CPKD childhood polycystic kidney disease

CPL criminal procedure law

CPM central pontine myelinolysis
chlorpheniramine maleate
Clinical Practice Model
continue present management
continuous passive motion
counts per minute
cyclophosphamide

CPmax peak serum concentration

CPMDI computerized pharmacokinetic model-driven drug infusion

CPmin trough serum concentration

CPMM constant passive motion machine

CPN chronic pyelonephritis

CPP cerebral perfusion pressure
chronic pelvic pain

CPPB continuous positive pressure breathing

CPPD calcium pyrophosphate dihydrate
cisplatin

CPPV continuous positive pressure ventilation
CPR cardiopulmonary resuscitation
tablet (French)
CPRAM controlled partial rebreathing anesthesia method
CPS cardiopulmonary support
chloroquine-pyremeth-aminesulfadoxine
clinical pharmacokinetic service
coagulase-positive staphylococci
complex partial seizures
CPT chest physio-therapy
child protection team
CPTH chronic post-traumatic headache
CPUE chest pain of unknown etiology
CPX complete physical examination
CPZ chlorpromazine
Compazine® (this is a dangerous abbreviation)
CR cardiac rehabilitation
cardiorespiratory
case reports
chief resident
closed reduction
colon resection
complete remission
contact record
controlled release
creamed
Cr chromium
C & R cystoscopy and retrograde
CR_1 first cranial nerve
CRA central retinal artery
chronic rheumatoid arthritis
colorectal anastomosis
CRAG cerebral radionuclide angiography
CRAMS Circulation, Respiration, Abdomen, Motor, and Speech
CRAO central retinal artery occlusion
CRBBB complete right bundle branch block
CRC child-resistant container
clinical research center
colorectal cancer
CR & C closed reduction and cast
CrCl creatinine clearance
CRD childhood rheumatic disease
chronic renal disease
chronic respiratory disease
cone-rod dystrophy
congenital rubella deafness
CREAT serum creatinine
CREST calcinosis, Raynaud's phenomenon, esophageal dysmotility, sclerodactyly, and telangiectasia
CRF chronic renal failure
corticotropin-releasing factor
CRI Cardiac Risk Index
catheter-related infection
chronic renal insufficiency
CRIE crossed radioimmuno-electrophoresis
crit. hematocrit
CRL crown rump length
CRM + cross-reacting material positive
CRNA Certified Registered Nurse Anesthetist
CRNI Certified Registered Nurse Intravenous
CRNP Certified Registered Nurse Practitioner
CRO cathode ray oscilloscope
CROS contralateral routing of signals
CRP chronic relapsing pancreatitis
coronary rehabilitation program

C-reactive protein
CRPD chronic restrictive pulmonary disease
CRPF chloroquine-resistant plasmodium falciparum
CRS catheter-related sepsis
Chinese restaurant syndrome
colon-rectal surgery
congenital rubella syndrome
CRST calcification, Raynaud's phenomenom, scleroderma, and telangiectasia
CRT cadaver renal transplant
cathode ray tube
central reaction time
copper reduction test
cranial radiation therapy
Cr Tr crutch training
CRTT Certified Respiratory Therapy Technician
CRTX cast removed take x-ray
CRU cardiac rehabilitation unit
clinical research unit
CRV central retinal vein
CRVF congestive right ventricular failure
CRVO central retinal vein occlusion
CRYST crystals
CS cat scratch
cervical spine
cesarean section
chest strap
cholesterol stone
cigarette smoker
clinical stage
close supervision
conjunctiva-sclera
consciousness
Cushing's syndrome
cycloserine
consultation
consultation service
C&S conjunctiva and sclera
culture and sensitivity
C/S cesarean section
culture and sensitivity
CSA controlled substance analogue
CsA cyclosporin
CSB caffeine sodium benzoate
Cheyne-Stokes breathing
CSB I & II Chemistry Screening Batteries I and II
CSBF coronary sinus blood flow
CSC cornea, sclera, and conjunctiva
CSCI continuous subcutaneous infusion
CSD cat scratch disease
C S&D cleaned, sutured, and dressed
CSE cross-section echocardiography
C sect. cesarean section
CSF cerebrospinal fluid
colony-stimulating factors
CSFP cerebrospinal fluid pressure
C-Sh chair shower
CSH carotid sinus hypersensitivity
chronic subdural hematoma
CSICU cardiac surgery intensive care unit
CSII continuous subcutaneous insulin infusion
CS IV clinical stage 4
CSLU chronic status leg ulcer
CSM carotid sinus massage
cerebrospinal meningitis
circulation, sensation, and movement
CSME cotton spot macular edema
CSNS carotid sinus nerve stimulation
CSO copied standing orders
CSOM chronic serous otitis media
chronic suppurative otitis media

CSP	cellulose sodium phosphate
CSR	central supply room
	Cheyne-Strokes respiration
	corrective septorhinoplasty
CSS	carotid sinus stimulation
	chewing, sucking, and swallowing
CST	cardiac stress test
	contraction stress test
	convulsive shock therapy
	cosyntropin stimulation test
	static compliance
CSU	cardiac surgery unit
	cardiac surveillance unit
	cardiovascular surgery unit
	casualty staging unit
	catheter specimen of urine
CT	calcitonin
	cardiothoracic
	carpal tunnel
	cervical traction
	chest tube
	circulation time
	clotting time
	coagulation time
	coated tablet
	compressed tablet
	computed tomography
	Coomb's test
	corneal thickness
	corneal transplant
	corrective therapy
	cytarabine and thioguanine
	cytoxic drug
CTA	catamenia (menses)
	clear to auscultation
C-TAB	cyanide tablet
CTAP	computed tomography during arterial portography
CTB	ceased to breathe
CTCL	cutaneous T-cell lymphoma
CT & DB	cough, turn & deep breath
CTD	carpal tunnel decompression
	chest tube drainage
	connective tissue disease
CTDW	continues to do well
CTF	Colorado tick fever
C/TG	cholesterol to triglyceride ratio
CTGA	complete transposition of the great arteries
CTH	clot to hold
CTI	certification of terminal illness
CTL	cervical, thoracic, and lumbar
	cytotoxic T lymphocytes
CTM	Chlor-Trimeton®
CT/MPR	computed tomography with multiplanar reconstructions
CTN	calcitonin
C & T N, BLE	color and temperature normal, both lower extremities
cTNM	clinical-diagnostic staging of cancer
CTP	comprehensive treatment plan
CTR	carpal tunnel release
CTS	carpal tunnel syndrome
CTSP	called to see patient
CTW	central terminal of Wilson
CTX	cyclophosphamide (Cytoxan®)
CTXN	contraction
CTZ	chemoreceptor trigger zone
	Co-Trimoxazole (sulfamethoxazole-trimethoprin)
Cu	copper
CU	cause unknown
CUC	chronic ulcerative colitis
CUD	cause undetermined
CUG	cystourethrogram
CUP	carcinoma of unknown primary (site)

CUPS carcinoma of unknown primary site
CUR curettage
CUS chronic undifferentiated schizophrenia
contact urticaria syndrome
CUSA Cavitron ultrasonic aspirator
CUT chronic undifferentiated type (schizophrenia)
CV cardiovascular
cell volume
cisplatin and etoposide
color vision
consonant vowel
CVA cerebrovascular accident
costovertebral angle
CVAH congenital virilizing adrenal hyperplasia
CVAT costovertebral angle tenderness
CVC central venous catheter
consonant vowel consonant
CVD collagen vascular disease
CVEB cisplatin, vinblastine, etoposide, and bleomycin
CVF cardiovascular failure
central visual field
cervicovaginal fluid
CVHD chronic valvular heart disease
CVI carboplatin, etoposide, ifosfamide, and mesna uroprotection
cerebrovascular insufficiency
continuous venous infusion
CVID common variable immune deficiency
CVN central venous nutrient
CVO central vein occlusion
conjugate diameter of pelvic inlet
CvO_2 mixed venous oxygen content
CVOR cardiovascular operating room
CVP central venous pressure
cyclophosphamide, vincristine and prednisone
CVPP lomustine, vinblastine, procarbazine, and prednisone
CVR cerebral vascular resistance
CVRI coronary vascular resistance index
CVS cardiovascular surgery
chorionic villi sampling
clean voided specimen
CVSU cardiovascular specialty unit
CVUG cysto-void urethrogram
CW careful watch
chest wall
clockwise
compare with
C/W consistent with
crutch walking
CWD cell wall defective
CWE cottonwool exudates
CWMS color, warmth, movement, and sensation
CWP childbirth without pain
coal worker's pneumoconiosis
CWS comfortable walking speed
cotton wool spots
Cx cancel
cervix
culture
cylinder axis
CxMT cervical motion tenderness
CXR chest x-ray
CXTX cervical traction
CY cyclophosphamide
CyA cyclosporine
CyADIC cyclophosphamide, doxorubicin, and dacarbazine

Cyclo C cyclocytidine HCl
CYL cylinder
CYSTO cystogram
cystoscopy
CYT cyclophosphamide
CYVA DIC cyclophosphamide, vincristine, adriamycin, and dacarbazine
CZI crystalline zinc insulin (regular insulin)
CZN chlorzotocin

D

D cholecalciferol
daughter
day
dead
dextrose
diarrhea
diastole
diopter
distal
divorced
D_1, D_2 dorsal vertebra #1, #2
D50 50% dextrose injection
2/d twice a day (this is a dangerous abbreviation)
2 D two-dimensional
3-D three-dimensional
DA degenerative arthritis
delivery awareness
diagnostic arthroscopy
direct admission
direct agglutination
dopamine
drug addict
drug aerosol
D/A discharge and advise
DA/A drug/alcohol addiction
DAB days after birth
DAC disabled adult child
Division of Ambulatory Care
DACL Depression Adjective Checklists
DACT dactinomycin
DAD diffuse alveolar damage
dispense as directed
drug administration device
DAE diving air embolism
DAG dianhydrogalactitol
DAH disordered action of the heart
DAI diffuse axonal injury
DAL drug analysis laboratory
DAM diacetylmonoxine
DANA drug induced antinuclear antibodies
DAP draw a person
diabetes-associated peptide
DAR daily affective rhythm
DARP drug abuse rehabilitation program
drug abuse reporting program
DAS developmental apraxia of speech
died at scene
DAT daunorubicin, cytaribine, (ARA-C), and thioguanine
dementia of the Alzheimer type
diet as tolerated
diphtheria antitoxin
direct agglutination test
direct antiglobulin test
DAW dispense as written
dB decibel
DB date of birth
deep breathe
direct bilirubin
double blind
DB & C deep breathing and coughing
DBD milolactol (dibromodulicitol)
DBE deep breathing exercise
DBED penicillin G benzathine
DBI® phenformin HCl
DBIL direct bilirubin
DBP diastolic blood pressure
DBQ debrisoquin
DBS diminished breath sounds
DBZ dibenzamine

DC	daunorubicin and cytarabine
	Doctor of Chiropractic
D&C	dilation and curettage
	direct and consensual
d/c, DC	decrease
	diagonal conjugate
	direct Coombs (test)
	discharged
	discontinue
DC65®	Darvon Compound 65®
DCA	sodium dichloroacetate
DCAG	double coronary artery graft
DCBE	double contrast barium enema
DCC	day care center
DCCF	dural carotid-cavernous fistula
DCE	delayed contrast-enhancement
	designated compensable event
DCFS	Department of Children and Family Services
DCH	delayed cutaneous hypersensitivity
DCIS	ductal carcinoma *in situ*
DCMXT	dichloromethotrexate
DCN	Darvocet N®
DCNU	chlorozotocin
DCO	diffusing capacity of carbon monoxide
DCP®	calcium phosphate, dibasic
DCPM	daunorubicin, cytarabine, prednisolone, and mercaptopurine
DCPN	direction-changing positional nystagmus
DCR	dacryocystorhinostomy
	delayed cutaneous reaction
DCS	decompression sickness
DCSA	double contrast shoulder arthrography
DCT	daunorubicin, cytarabine, and thioguanine
	deep chest therapy
	direct (antiglobulin) Coombs test
DCTM	delay computer tomographic myelography
DCYS	Department of Children and Youth Services
DD	dependent drainage
	dialysis dementia
	died of the disease
	differential diagnosis
	discharge diagnosis
	down drain
	dry dressing
	Duchenne's dystrophy
D→D	discharge to duty
D & D	diarrhea and dehydration
DDA	dideoxyadenosine
DDAVP®	desmopressin acetate
DDC	dideoxycytidine
DDD	defined daily doses
	degenerative disc disease
	fully automatic pacing
DDGB	double-dose gallbladder (test)
DDHT	double dissociated hypertropia
DDI	dideoxyinosine
DDP	cisplatin
DDS	dialysis disequilibrium syndrome
	doctor of dental surgery
	double decidual sac (sign)
	4, 4-diaminodiphenylsulfone (dapsone)
DDST	Denver Development Screening Test
DDT	chlorophenothane
DDx	differential diagnosis
D_5E_{48}	5% Dextrose and Electrolyte 48
D_5E_{75}	5% Dextrose and Electrolyte 75
2DE	two dimensional echocardiography
D&E	dilation and evacuation
DEA#	Drug Enforcement Administration number

(physician's Federal narcotic number)

DEC decrease
diethylcarbamazine

DECAFS Department of Children and Family Services

DECEL deceleration

decub decubitus

DEET diethyltoluamide

DEF decayed, extracted, or filled
defecation
deficiency

degen degenerative

del delivery, delivered

DEP ST SEG depressed ST segment

DER disulfiram-ethanol reaction

DERM dermatology

DES diethylstilbestrol
diffuse esophageal spasm
disequilibrium syndrome

DESAT desaturation

DET diethyltryptamine

DEV deviation
duck embryo vaccine

DEVR dominant exudative vitreoretinopathy

dex. dexter (right)

DF decayed and filled
degree of freedom
dengue fever
diabetic father
diastolic filling
dorsiflexion
drug free
dye free

DFA diet for age
difficulty falling asleep
direct fluorescent antibody

DFD defined formula diets

DFE distal femoral epiphysis

DFG direct forward gaze

DFI disease-free interval

DFM decreased fetal movement

DFMC daily fetal movement count

DFMO eflornithine (difluoromethylorithine)

DFMR daily fetal movement record

DFO deferoxamine

DFOM deferoxamine

DFP diastolic filling period
isoflurophate (diisopropyl flurophosphate)

DFR diabetic floor routine

DFRC deglycerolized frozen red cells

DFS disease-free survival

DFU dead fetus in uterus

DFW Dexide face wash

DGE delayed gastric emptying

DGI disseminated gonococcal infection

DGM ductal glandular mastectomy

DH delayed hypersensitivity
dermatitis herpetiformis
developmental history
diaphragmatic hernia

DHA dihydroxyacetone
docosahexaenoic acid

DHAD mitoxanthrone HCl

DHBV duck hepatitis B virus

DHE 45® dihydroergotamine mesylate

DHEA dehydroepiandrosterone

DHEAS dehydroepiandrosterone sulfate

DHF dengue hemorrhagic fever

DHFR dihydrofolate reductase

DHL diffuse histocytic lymphoma

DHPG ganciclovir

DHPR erythrocyte dihydropteridine reductase

DHS Department of Human Services
duration of hospital stay
dynamic hip screw

DHST delayed hypersensitivity test

DHT dihydrotachysterol
dissociated hypertropia

DI (Beck) Depression Inventory

	date of injury
	Debrix Index
	detrusor instability
	diabetes insipidus
	diagnostic imaging
	drug interactions
D&I	dry and intact
diag.	diagnosis
DIAS BP	diastolic blood pressure
Diath SW	diathermy short wave
DIAZ	diazepam
DIB	disability insurance benefits
DIC	dacarbazine
	disseminated intravascular coagulation
	drug information center
DID	delayed ischemia deficit
DIE	die in emergency department
DIFF	differential blood count
DIG	digoxin (this is a dangerous abbreviation)
DIH	died in hospital
DIJOA	dominantly inherited juvenile optic atrophy
DIL	dilute
	drug-induced lupus
DILD	diffuse infiltrative lung disease
DILE	drug induced lupus erythematosus
DIM	diminish
DIMOAD	diabetes insipidus, diabetes mellitus, optic atrophy, and deafness
DIMS	disorder of initiating and maintaining sleep
DIP	desquamative interstitial pneumonia
	distal interphalangeal
	drip infusion pyelogram
	drug-induced parkinsonism
DIPJ	distal interphalangeal joint
DIR	directions
DIS	Diagnostic Interview Schedule (questionnaire)
	dislocation
disch.	discharge
DISH	diffuse idiopathic skeletal hyperostosis
D_5ISOM	5% Dextrose and Isolyte M
D_5ISOP	5% Dextrose and Isolyte P
dist.	distal
	distilled
DIT	diiodotyrosine
	drug-induced thrombocytopenia
DIV	double inlet ventricle
DIVA	digital intravenous angiography
DJD	degenerative joint disease
DK	dark
	diabetic ketoacidosis
	diseased kidney
DKA	diabetic ketoacidosis
	didn't keep appointment
dl	deciliter (100 mL)
DL	danger list
	deciliter
	diagnostic laparoscopy
	direct laryngoscopy
	drug level
D_L	maximal diffusing capacity
DLB	direct laryngoscopy and bronchoscopy
DLC	double lumen catheter
DLCO sb	diffuse capacity of carbon monoxide, single breath
DLE	discoid lupus erythematosus
DLF	digitalis-like factor
DLIF	digoxin-like immunoreactive factors
DLIS	digoxin-like immunoreactive substance
DLMP	date of last menstrual period
DLNMP	date of last normal menstrual period
D5LR	dextrose 5% in lactated Ringer's injection
DLS	daily living skills
DM	dermatomyositis

	dextromethorphan
	diabetes mellitus
	diabetic mother
	diastolic murmur
DMAD	disease-modifying antirheumatic drug
DMARD	disease modifying antirheumatic drug
DMBA	dimethylbenzantracene
DMC	dactinomycin, methotrexate, and cyclophosphamide
DMD	Doctor of Dental Medicine
	Duchenne's muscular dystrophy
DME	durable medical equipment
DMF	decayed, missing or filled
DMI	desipramine
	diaphragmatic myocardial infarction
DMKA	diabetes mellitus ketoacidosis
DMO	dimethadone
DMOOC	diabetes mellitus out of control
DMSA	dimercaptosuccinic acid
DMSO	dimethyl sulfoxide
DMT	dimethyltryptamine
DMV	Doctor of Veterinary Medicine
DMX	diathermy, massage and exercise
DN	diabetic nephropathy
	dicrotic notch
	down
	dysplastic nevus
D & N	distance and near (vision)
D_5 1/2NS	dextrose 5% in 0.45% sodium chloride injection
DNA	deoxyribonucleic acid
	did not answer
	did not attend
	does not apply
DNCB	dinitrochlorobenzene
DNC	did not come
DND	died a natural death
DNI	do not intubate
DNKA	did not keep appointment
DNP	dinitrophenylhydrazine
	do not publish
DNR	daunorubicin
	did not respond
	do not report
	do not resuscitate
	dorsal nerve root
DNS	deviated nasal septum
	doctor did not see patient
	do not show
	dysplastic nevus syndrome
D_5NSS	5% dextrose in normal saline solution
DNT	did not test
DO	diet order
	distocclusal
	Doctor of Osteopathy
	doctor's order
D/O	disorder
DOA	date of admission
	dead on arrival
	duration of action
DOA-DRA	dead on arrival despite resuscitative attempts
DOB	dangle out of bed
	date of birth
	dobutamine
	doctor's order book
DOC	diabetes out of control
	died of other causes
	drug of choice
DOCA	desoxycorticosterone acetate
DOD	date of death
DOE	dyspnea on exertion
DOES	disorder of excessive somnolence
DOH	Department of Health
DOI	date of injury
DOL #2	second day of life
DOLV	double outlet left ventricle
DON	Director of Nursing
DOP	dopamine
DORV	double-outlet right ventricle
DORx	date of treatment
DOSS	docusate sodium (dioctyl sodium sulfosuccinate)

DOT	date of transcription
	date of transfer
	died on table
	Doppler ophthalmic test
DOX	doxorubicin
doz	dozen
DP	diastolic pressure
	disability pension
	discharge planning
	dorsalis pedis (pulse)
DPA	Department of Public Assistance
DPB	days postburn
DPC	delayed primary closure
	discharge planning coordinator
DPDL	diffuse poorly differentiated lymphocytic lymphoma
2,3-DPG	2,3-diphosphoglyceric acid
DPH	Department of Public Health
	diphenhydramine
	Doctor of Public Health
	phenytoin (diphenylhydantoin)
DPL	diagnostic peritoneal lavage
DPM	distintegrations per minute (dpm)
	Doctor of Podiatric Medicine
	drops per minute
DPT	Demerol®, Phenergan®, and Thorazine® (this is a dangerous abbreviation)
	diphtheria, pertussis, and tetanus (immunization)
	Driver Performance Test
DPTPM	diphtheria, pertussis, tetanus, poliomyelitis, and measles
DPU	delayed pressure urticaria
DPUD	duodenal peptic ulcer disease
Dr.	doctor
DR	delivery room
	diabetic retinopathy
	diagnostic radiology
	diurnal rhythm
DRA	drug-related admissions
DRE	digital rectal examination
DRESS	depth resolved surface coil spectroscopy
DREZ	dorsal root entry zone
DRG	diagnosis-related groups
DRGE	drainage
drI	Discharge Readiness Index
DRS	Duane's retraction syndrome
DRSG	dressing
DRUB	drug screen-blood
DS	deep sleep
	dextrose stick
	discharge summary
	disoriented
	double strength
	Down's syndrome
D/S	5% dextrose and 0.9% sodium chloride injection
D&S	diagnostic and surgical
	dilation and suction
D5S	dextrose 5% in 0.9% sodium chloride (saline)
DSA	(angiocardiography)
	digital subtraction angiography
DSD	discharge summary dictated
	dry sterile dressing
DSDB	direct self-destructive behavior
dsg	dressing
DSI	deep shock insulin
	Depression Status Inventory
DSM	drink skim milk
DSM III	Diagnostic & Statistical Manual, 3rd Edition
DSP	digital signal processor
DSRF	drainage subretinal fluid
DSS	dengue shock syndrome
	Disability Status Scale
	docusate sodium
DST	dexamethasone

suppression test
donor specific transfusion

DSU day surgery unit

DSV digital subtraction ventriculography

DSWI deep surgical wound infection

DT delirium tremens
dietetic technician
diphtheria tetanus
diphtheria toxoid
discharge tomorrow

D&T diagnosis and treatment

DTBC tubocurarine (d-tubocurarine)

DTC day treatment center

DTD #30 dispense 30 such doses

DTH delayed-type hypersensitivity

DTIC dacarbazine

DTPA pentetic acid (diethylenetriaminepentaacetic acid)

DTR deep tendon reflexes

DTs delirium tremens

DTS donor specific transfusion

DTT diphtheria tetanus toxoid
dithiothreitol

DTUS diathermy, traction, and ultrasound

DTV due to void

DTX detoxification

DU diabetic urine
diagnosis undetermined
duodenal ulcer
duroxide uptake

DUB Dubowitz (score)
dysfunctional uterine bleeding

DUI driving under the influence

DUID driving under the influence of drugs

DUNHL diffuse undifferentiated non-Hodgkins lymphoma

DUR drug use review
duration

DV distance vision

D&V diarrhea and vomiting

DVA vindesine

DVC direct visualization of vocal cords

DVD dissociated vertical deviation

DVI atrioventricular sequential pacing
digital vascular imaging

DVIU direct vision internal urethrotomy

DVM Doctor of Veterinary Medicine

DVP cyclophosphamide, vincristine, and prednisone

DVP-Asp daunorubicin, vincristine, prednisone, and asparaginase

DVPA daunorubicin, vincristine, prednisone, and asparaginase

DVR Division of Vocational Rehabilitation
double valve replacement

DVSA digital venous subtraction angiography

DVT deep vein thrombosis

D_5W 5% dextrose (in water) injection

DW deionized water
dextrose in water
distilled water

5 DW 5% dextrose (in water) injection

DWDL diffuse well differentiated lymphocytic lymphoma

DWI driving while intoxicated

DWRT delayed work recall test

Dx diagnosis

DXM dexamethasone

DXRT deep x-ray therapy

DYF drag your feet (author's note: see you in court)

DZ diazepam
disease
dizygotic
dozen

E

E	edema engorged eosinophil expired eye
E2	estradiol
E3	estriol
4E	4 plus edema
E →A	say E,E,E, comes out as A,A,A upon auscultation of lung showing consolidation
EA	elbow aspiration enteral alimentation
E&A	evaluate and advise
EAA	electrothermal atomic absorption essential amino acids
EAC	external auditory canal
EACA	aminocaproic acid
EAHF	eczema, allergy, hay, and fever
EAM	external auditory meatus
EAP	Employment Assistance Programs
EAS	external anal sphincter
EAST	external rotation, abduction stress test
EAT	ectopic atrial tachycardia
EAU	experimental autoimmune uveitis
EB	epidermolysis bullosa Epstein-Barr
EBA	epidermolysis bullosa acquisita
EBAB	equal breath sounds bilaterally
EBC	esophageal balloon catheter
EBF	erythroblastosis fetalis
EBL	estimated blood loss
EBM	expressed breast milk
EBS	epidermolysis bullosa
EBV	Epstein-Barr virus
EC	ejection click enteric coated *Escherichia coli* extracellular eyes closed
ECA	ethacrynic acid external carotid artery
ECBD	exploration of common bile duct
ECC	emergency cardiac care endocervical curettage external cardiac compression
ECCE	extracapsular cataract extraction
ECD	endocardial cushion defect
ECEMG	evoked compound electromyography
ECF	extended care facility extracellular fluid
ECG	electrocardiogram
ECHINO	echinocyte
ECHO	echocardiogram enterocytopathogenic human orphan (virus) etoposide, cyclophosphamide, Adriamycin®, and vincristine
ECHO/NV	echocardiography/radionuclide ventriculography
ECL	extend of cerebral lesion extracapillary lesions
ECM	erythema chronicum migrans
ECMO	extracorporeal membrane oxygenation (oxygenator)
ECN	extended care nursery
ECOG	Eastern Cooperative Oncology Group
ECPD	external counterpressure device
ECR	emergency chemical restraint
ECRL	extensor carpi radialis longus
ECS	electrocerebral silence
ECT	electroconvulsive therapy emission computed tomography

	enhanced computer tomography
ECU	extensor carpi ulnaris
ECW	extracellular water
ED	elbow disarticulation
	emergency department
	epidural
ED_{50}	median effective dose
EDAP	Emergency Department Approved for Pediatrics
EDAX	energy-dispersive analysis of x-rays
EDB	ethylene dibromide
EDC	effective dynamic compliance
	electrodesiccation and curettage
	end diastolic counts
	estimated date of conception
	estimated date of confinement
	extensor digitorium communis
EDD	expected date of delivery
EDF	elongation, derotation, and flexion
EDH	epidural hematoma
EDM	early diastolic murmur
EDP	emergency department physician
	end diastolic pressure
EDR	edrophonium
EDRF	endothelium derived relaxing factor
EDS	Ehlers-Danlos syndrome
EDTA	edetic acid (ethylenedinitrilo tetraacetic acid)
EDV	end-diastolic volume
EE	end to end
	equine encephalitis
	external ear
	eye and ear
EEA	elemental enteral alimentation
	end-to-end anastomosis
EEE	Eastern equine encephalomyelitis
	edema, erythema, and exudate
	external eye examination
EEG	electroencephalogram
EENT	eyes, ears, nose, and throat
EES®	erythromycin ethylsuccinate
EF	ejection fraction
	endurance factor
	extended-field (radiotherapy)
EFAD	essential fatty acid deficiency
EFE	endocardial fibroelastosis
EFHBM	eosinophilic fibrohistiocytic lesion of bone marrow
EFM	electronic fetal monitor(ing)
	external fetal monitoring
EFW	estimated fetal weight
EF/WM	ejection fraction/wall motion
e.g.	for example
EGA	estimated gestational age
EGBUS	external genitalia, Bartholin, urethral, and Skene's glands
EGD	esophagogastroduodenoscopy
EGF	epidermal growth factor
EGG	electrogastrography
EGL	eosinophilic granuloma of the lung
EGTA	esophageal gastric tube airway
EH	educationally handicapped
	enlarged heart
	essential hypertension
	extramedullary hematopoiesis
EHDA	etidronate sodium
EHB	elevate head of bed
EHE	epithelioid hemangioendothelioma
EHF	epidemic hemorrhagic fever
EHL	electrohydraulic lithotripsy
	extensor hallucis longus
E & I	endocrine and infertility

EIA	enzyme immunoassay exercise induced asthma
EIAB	extracranial-intracranial arterial bypass
EIB	exercise induced bronchospasm
EID	electroimmunodiffusion electronic infusion device
EIP	end-inspiratory pressure
EIS	endoscopic injection scleropathy
EJ	elbow jerk external jugular
EKC	epidemic keratoconjuctivitis
EKG	electrocardiogram
EKO	echoencephalogram
EKY	electrokymogram
E-L	external lids
ELF	elective low forceps
ELH	endolymphatic hydrops
ELI	endomyocardial lymphocytic infiltrates
ELISA	enzyme-linked immunosorbent assay
Elix	elixir
ELLIP	ellipotocytosis
ELOP	estimated length of program
ELOS	estimated length of stay
ELP	electrophoresis
ELPS	excessive lateral pressure syndrome
ELS	Eaton-Lambert syndrome
EM	early memory ejection murmur electron microscope emmetropia erythema migrans erythema multiforme extensive metabolizers
EMA-CO	etoposide, methotrexate, dactinomycin, and leucovorin
EMB	endometrial biopsy endomyocardial biopsy ethambutol
EMC	encephalomyocarditis
EMD	electromechanical dissociation
EMF	erythrocyte maturation factor evaporated milk formula
EMG	electromyograph emergency essential monoclonal gammopathy
EMIC	emergency maternity and infant care
E-MICR	electron microscopy
EMIT	enzyme multiplied immunoassay technique
EMLB	erythromycin lactobionate
EMMW	extended mandatory minute ventilation
EMR	educable mentally retarded emergency mechanical restraint empty, measure, and record
EMS	early morning stiffness emergency medical services eosinophilia myalgia syndrome
EMT	emergency medical technician
EMV	eye, motor, verbal (grading for Glasgow coma scale)
EMVC	early mitral valve closure
EMW	electromagnetic waves
EN	enteral nutrition erythema nodosum
ENA	extractable nuclear antigen
ENC	encourage
ENDO	endodontia endoscopy endotracheal
ENF	Enfamil®
ENG	electronystagmogram engorged
ENL	erythema nodosum leprosum
ENP	extractable nucleoprotein
ENT	ears, nose, throat
EO	elbow orthosis eosinophilia

	ethylene oxide
	eyes open
EOA	esophageal obturator airway
	examine, opinion, and advice
EOC	enema of choice
EOD	every other day (this is a dangerous abbreviation)
EOG	electro-oculogram
	Ethrane®, oxygen, and gas (nitrous oxide)
EOM	external otitis media
	extraocular movement
	extraocular muscles
EOMI	extraocular muscles intact
EORA	elderly onset rheumatoid arthritis
eos.	eosinophil
EP	ectopic pregnancy
	electrophysiologic
	elopement precaution
	endogenous pyrogen
	evoked potentials
E&P	estrogen and progesterone
EPA	eicosapentaenoic acid
EPB	extensor pollicis brevis
EPC	erosive prephloric changes
EPF	Enfamil Premature Formula®
EPEG	etoposide
EPI	epinephrine
	epitheloid cells
	exocrine pancreatic insufficiency
EPIS	episiotomy
epith.	epithelial
EPL	extensor pollicis longus
EPM	electronic pacemaker
EPO	erythropoietin
EPP	erythropoietic protoporphyria
EPR	electrophrenic respiration
	emergency physical restraint
EPS	electrophysiologic study
	extrapyramidal syndrome (symptom)
EPT®	early pregnancy test
EPTS	existed prior to service
ER	emergency room
	estrogen receptors
	external rotation
E & R	equal and reactive
	examination and report
ER+	estrogen receptor-positive
ERA	estrogen receptor assay
	evoked response audiometry
ERCP	endoscopic retrograde cholangiopancreatography
ERD	early retirement with disability
ERE	external rotation in extension
ERF	external rotation in flexion
ERFC	erythrocyte rosette forming cells
ERG	electroretinogram
ERL	effective refractory length
ERP	emergency room physician
	endoscopic retrograde pancreatography
	event-related potentials
	estrogen receptor protein
ERPF	effective renal plasma flow
ERT	estrogen replacement therapy
ERV	expiratory reserve volume
ES	emergency service
	end-to-side
	ex-smoker
ESA	end-to-side anastomosis
ESAP	evoked sensory (nerve) action potention
ESC	end systolic counts
ESD	Emergency Services Department
	esophagus, stomach, and duodenum
ESF	external skeletal fixation
ESLD	end-stage liver disease
ESM	ejection systolic murmur
ESO	esophagus
ESP	end systolic pressure

	especially
	extrasensory perception
ESR	erythrocyte sedimentation rate
ESRD	end-stage renal disease
ess.	essential
EST	electroshock therapy
	exercise stress test
ESWL	extracorporeal shockwave lithotripsy
ET	ejection time
	endotracheal
	enterostomal therapy (therapist)
	esotropia
	essential thrombocythemia
	essential tremor
	eustachian tube
	exchange transfusion
	exercise treadmill
et	and
E(T)	intermittent esotropia
ETA	endotracheal airway
	ethionamide
et al	and others
ETC	and so forth
	estimated time of conception
$ETCO_2$	end tidal carbon dioxide
ETD	eustachian tube dysfunction
ETE	end-to-end
ETF	eustachian tubal function
ETH	elixir terpin hydrate
	ethanol
	Ethrane®
ETHc̄C	elixir terpin hydrate with codeine
ETI	ejective time index
ETKTM	every test known to man
ETO	estimated time of ovulation
	ethylene oxide
	eustachian tube obstruction
ETOH	alcohol
	alcoholic
ETOP	elective termination of pregnancy
ETP	elective termination of pregnancy
ETS	end-to-side
ETT	endotracheal tube
	exercise tolerance test
ETU	emergency and trauma unit
	emergency treatment unit
EU	esophageal ulcer
	etiology unknown
	excretory urography
EUA	examine under anesthesia
EUCD	emotionally unstable character disorder
EUG	extrauterine gestation
EUM	external urethral meatus
EUP	extrauterine pregnancy
EUS	external urethral sphincter
EV	esophageal varices
EVAC	evacuation
eval	evaluate
EVE	evening
EVS	endoscopic variceal sclerosis
ew	elsewhere
EWB	estrogen withdrawal bleeding
EWHO	elbow-wrist-hand orthosis
EWSCLs	extended-wear soft contact lenses
EWT	erupted wisdom teeth
ex	examined
	excision
	exercise
exam.	examination
EXEF	exercise ejection fraction
EXP	experienced
	exploration
	expose
expect	expectorant
exp. lap.	exploratory laparotomy
EXT	extension
	external
	extract
	extraction
Ext mon	external monitor
extrav	extravasation
ext. rot.	external rotation
EXTUB	extubation
EX U	excretory urogram

F

F	facial
	Fahrenheit
	fair
	fasting
	father
	female
	finger
	firm
	flow
	fluoride
	French
	fundi
F/	full upper denture
/F	full lower denture
(F)	final
F_1	offspring from the first generation
F_2	offspring from the second generation
F II	factor II (two)
F VIII	factor VIII (8)
FA	femoral artery
	folic acid
	forearm
FAAP	family assessment adjustment pass
FAA SOL	formalin, acetic, and alcohol solution
FAAN	Fellow of the American Academy of Nursing
FAAP	Fellow of the American Academy of Pediatrics
FAB	digoxin immune Fab (Digibind®)
	French-American-British Cooperative group
	functional arm brace
FABER	full abduction and external rotation
FABF	femoral artery blood flow
FAC	fluorouracil, Adriamycin®, and cyclophosphamide
	fractional area concentration
FACA	Fellow of the American College of Anaesthetists
FACAG	Fellow of the American College of Angiology
FACAL	Fellow of the American College of Allergists
FACAN	Fellow of the American College of Anesthesiologists
FACAS	Fellow of the American College of Abdominal Surgeons
FACC	Fellow of the American College of Cardiology
FACCP	Fellow of the American College of Chest Physicians
FACCPC	Fellow of the American College of Clinical Pharmacology & Chemotherapy
FACD	Fellow of the American College of Dentists
FACEM	Fellow of the American College of Emergency Medicine
FACEP	Fellow of the American College of Emergency Physicians
FACGE	Fellow of the American College of Gastroenterology
FACH	forceps to after-coming head
FACLM	Fellow of the American College of Legal Medicine
FACN	Fellow of the American College of Nutrition
FACNP	Fellow of the American College of Neuro-psychopharmacology
FACOG	Fellow of the American College of Obstetricians & Gynecologists
FACOS	Fellow of the American College of Orthopedic Surgeons
FACP	Fellow of the American College of Physicians
FACPRM	Fellow of the American

College of Preventive Medicine

FACR Fellow of the American College of Radiology

FACS Fellow of the American College of Surgeons

FACSM Fellow of the American College of Sports Medicine

FAD Family Accessment Device

FAGA full-term appropriate for gestational age

FAI functional assessment inventory

FALL fallopian

FAM family
fluorouracil, Adriamycin, and mitomycin

FAMA fluorescent antibody to membrane antigen

FAME fluorouracil, doxorubicin, and methyl CCNU

FANA fluorescent antinuclear antibody

FAP familial adenomatous polyposis
familial amyloid polyneuropathy
femoral artery pressure
fibrillating action potential

FAS fetal alcohol syndrome

FASHP Fellow of the American Society of Hospital Pharmacists

FAST fluorescent allergo sorbent technique

FAT fluorescent antibody test

FB fasting blood (sugar)
finger breadth
foreign body

F/B forward bending

FBC full blood count

FBD fibrocystic breast disease
functional bowel disease

FBF forearm blood flow

FBG foreign-body-type granulomata

FBH hydroxybutyric dehydrogenase

FBL fecal blood loss

FBRCM fingerbreadth below right costal margin

FBS fasting blood sugar
fetal bovine serum

FBU fingers below umbilicus

FBW fasting blood work

FC family conference
febrile convulsions
financial class
finger clubbing
finger counting
flucytosine
foley catheter
foster care
functional capacity

5-FC flucytosine

FC fever, chills
finger clubbing
function capacity
functional class

F + C flare and cells

F & C foam and condom

F. cath. foley catheter

FCC familial colonic cancer
femoral cerebral catheter
follicular center cells
fracture compound comminuted

FCCL follicular center cell lymphoma

FCD fibrocystic disease

FCDB fibrocystic disease of the breast

FCE fluorouracil, cisplatin, and etoposide

FCH familial combined hyperlipidemia

FCHL familial combined hyperlipemia

F-CL fluorouracil and calcium leucovorin

FCMC family centered maternity care

FCMD Fukiyama's congenital muscular dystrophy

FCMN family centered maternity nursing

FCR flexor carpi radialis
FCRB flexor carpi radialis brevis
FCSNVD fever, chills, sweating, nausea, vomiting, and diarrhea
FCU flexor carpi ulnaris
FD familial dysautonomia
fetal demise
focal distance
forceps delivery
full denture
F & D fixed and dilated
FDA Food and Drug Administration
fronto-dextra anterior
FDBL fecal daily blood loss
FDG feeding
fluorine-18-labeled deoxyglucose
FDGS feedings
FDIU fetal death in utero
FDLMP first day of last menstrual period
FDM fetus of diabetic mother
FDP fibrin-degradation products
flexor digitorum profundus
FDS flexor digitorum superficialis
for duration of stay
Fe female
iron
FEC fluorouracil, etoposide, and cisplatin
forced expiratory capacity
FECG fetal electrocardiogram
FEF forced expiratory flow rate
$FEF_{25\%-75\%}$ forced expiratory flow during the middle half of the forced vital capacity
FEF_{x-y} forced expiratory flow between two designated volume points in the forced vital capacity
FEL familial erythrophagocytic lymphohistiocytosis
FeLV feline leukemia virus
FEM femoral
Fem-pop femoral popliteal (bypass)
FEN fluid, electrolytes, and nutrition
FENa fractional extraction of sodium
FEP free erythrocyte protoporphorin
FES fat embolism syndrome
functional electrical stimulation
$FeSO_4$ ferrous sulfate
FEUO for external use only
FEV_1 forced expiratory volume in one second
FF fat free
fecal frequency
filtration fraction
finger to finger
flat feet
force fluids
foster father
fundus firm
F&F fixes and follows
FFA free fatty acid
FFB flexible fiberoptic bronchoscopy
FFD fat-free diet
FFI fast food intake
FFM fat-free mass
five finger movement
FFP fresh frozen plasma
FFS flexible fiberoptic sigmoidoscopy
FFT fast-Fourier transforms
FFTP first full-term pregnancy
FG fibrin glue
FGP fundic gland polyps
FH family history
fetal head
fetal heart
fundal height
FHF fulminant hepatic failure
FHH familial hypocalciuric hypercalcemia
fetal heart heard
FHI Fuch's heterochromic iridocyclitis
FHL flexor hallucis longus
FHNH fetal heart not heard

FHP family history positive
FHR fetal heart rate
FHS fetal heart sounds
fetal hydantoin syndrome
FHT fetal heart tone
$FiCO_2$ fraction of inspired carbon dioxide
FID father in delivery
FIF forced inspiratory flow
FIGLU formiminoglutamic acid
FIGO International Federation of Gynecology and Obstetrics
FIL father-in-law
FIM functional independence measure
FiO_2 fraction of inspired oxygen
FIPT periarteriolar transudate
FISP fast imaging with steady state precision
FITC fluorescein isothiocynate
FIVC forced inspiratory vital capacity
FJROM full joint range of motion
FJS finger joint size
FL fatty liver
fetal length
fluid
flutamide and leuprolide acetate
full liquids
FLASH fast low-angle shot
FLD fatty liver disease
fluid
flutamide and leuprolide acetate depot
FLGA full-term, large for gestational age
FLK funny looking kid (should never be used: unusual facial features, is a better expression)
FLS flashing lights and/ or scotoma
FLU A influenza A virus
FLW fasting laboratory work
FLZ flurazepam
FM face mask
fetal movements
F & M firm and midline (uterus)
FMC fetal movement count
FMD family medical doctor
fibromuscular dysplasia
foot and mouth disease
FME full mouth extraction
FMF familial Mediterranean fever
fetal movement felt
forced midexpiratory flow
FMG fine mesh gauze
foreign medical graduate
FMH family medical history
fibromuscular hyperplasia
FML® fluorometholone
FMN first malignant neoplasm
FMP fasting metabolic panel
first menstrual period
FMR fetal movement record
FMS fluorouracil, mitomycin, and streptozocin
full mouth series
FMV fluorouracil, methyl-CCNU, and vincristine
FMX full mouth x-ray
FN false negative
finger-to-nose
F to N finger to nose
FNA fine-needle aspiration
FNAB fine-needle aspiration biopsy
FNAC fine-needle aspiratory cytology
FNCJ fine needle catheter jejunostomy
FNF finger nose finger
FNH focal nodular hyperplasia
FNR false negative rate
FNS food and nutrition services
functional neuromuscular stimulation
FNT finger to nose test
FO foot orthosis
foreign object
fronto-occipital
FOB father of baby
fecal occult blood
feet out of bed

	fiberoptic bronchoscope
	foot of bed
FOBT	fecal occult blood test
FOC	father of child
	fluid of choice
	fronto-occipital circumference
FOD	free of disease
FOEB	feet over edge of bed
FOG	Fluothane®, oxygen and gas (nitrous oxide)
	full-on gain
FOI	flight of ideas
FOM	floor of mouth
FOMi	fluorouracil, Oncovin, (vincristine), and mitomycin
FOOB	fell out of bed
FOOSH	fell on outstretched hand
FOV	field of view
FP	false positive
	family planning
	family practice
	flat plate
	food poisoning
	frozen plasma
F-P	femoral popliteal
fpA	fibrinopeptide A
F.P.A.L.	fullterm, premature, abortion, living
FPB	flexor pollicis brevis
FPC	familial polyposis coli
	family practice center
FPD	feto-pelvic disproportion
	fixed partial denture
FPG	fasting plasma glucose
FPHx	family psychiatric history
FPIA	fluorescence-polarization immunoassay
FPL	flexor pollicis longus
FPM	full passive movements
FPNA	first-pass nuclear angiocardiography
FPZ	fluphenazine
FPZ-D	fluphenazine decanoate
FR	father
	Father (priest)
	flow rate
	fluid restriction
F & R	force & rhythm (pulse)
FRACTS	fractional urines
FRC	functional residual capacity
FRE	flow-related enhancement
FRF	filtration replacement fluid
FRJM	full range of joint movement
FROM	full range of motion
FS	fingerstick
	flexible sigmoidoscopy
	frozen section
	full strength
F & S	full and soft
FSALO	Fletcher suite after loading ovoids
FSALT	Fletcher suite after loading tandem
FSB	fetal scalp blood
FSBM	full strength breast milk
FSC	fracture, simple, and complete
FSD	fracture, simple, depressed
FSE	fetal scalp electrode
FSG	focal & segmental glomerulosclerosis
FSGA	full-term, small for gestational age
FSGS	focal segmental glomerulosclerosis
FSH	facioscapulohumeral
	follicle stimulating hormone
FSHMD	facioscapulohumeral muscular dystrophy
FSIQ	Full-Scale Intelligence Quotient
F-SM/C	fungus, smear and culture
FSP	fibrin split products
FSS	French steel sound (dilated to #24FSS)
	full scale score
FSW	field service worker
FT	family therapy
	filling time
	finger tip
	follow through
	foot (ft)
	full term

FT_3	free triiodorhyroxine
FT_4	free thyroxine
F_3T	trifluridine
FTA	fluorescent titer antibody fluorescent treponemal antibody
FTB	fingertip blood
FTBD	full-term born dead
FTD	failure to descend
FTE	full-time equivalent
FTFTN	finger-to-finger-to-nose
FTG	full thickness graft
FTI	free thyroxine index
FTKA	failed to keep appointment
FTLB	full-term living birth
FTLFC	full term living female child
FTLMC	full term living male child
FTN	finger-to-nose full term nursery
FTNB	full-term newborn
FTND	full-term normal delivery
FTNSD	full-term, normal, spontaneous delivery
FTP	failure to progress
FTR	for the record
FTSG	full-thickness skin graft
FTT	failure to thrive
F & U	flanks and upper quadrants
F/U	follow-up fundus at umbilicus
F ↑U	fingers above umbilicus
F ↓U	fingers below umbilicus
5-FU	fluorouracil
FUB	function uterine bleeding
FUDR®	floxuridine
FUN	follow-up note
FUNG-C	fungus culture
FUNG-S	fungus smear
FUO	fever of undetermined origin
FUOV	follow-up office visit
FUS	fusion
FV	femoral vein
FVC	filled voiding flow rate forced vital capacity
FVH	focal vascular headache
FVL	femoral vein ligation
	flow volume loop
F waves	fibrillatory waves flutter waves
FWB	full weight bearing
FWW	front wheel walker
Fx	fractional urine fracture
Fx-dis	fracture-dislocation
FXN	function
FXR	fracture
FYI	for your information

G

G	gallop gauge good grade gram (g) gravida
G +	Gram-positive
G −	Gram-negative
G1–4	grade 1–4
G-11	hexachlorophene
GA	Gamblers Anonymous gastric analysis general anesthesia general appearance gestational age ginger ale glucose/acetone
Ga	gallium
GABA	gamma-aminobutyric acid
GABHS	group A beta hemolytic streptococci
GAG	glycosaminoglycan
Gal	gallon
G'ale	ginger ale
GALI-PUT	galactose-1-phosphate uridye transferase enzyme
GAS	general adaption syndrome Glasgow Assessment Schedule Global Assessment Scale group *A streptococcus*
Gas Anal F&T	gastric analysis, free and total
Ga scan	gallium scan

Gastroc	gastrocnemius
GAT	group adjustment therapy
GATB	General Aptitude Test Battery
GAU	geriatric assessment unit
Gaw	airway conductance
GB	gallbladder
G & B	good and bad
GBA	ganglionic-blocking agent
GBBS	group B beta hemolytic streptococcus
GBE	*Ginkgo biloba* extract
GBH	gamma benzene hexachloride (lindane)
GBM	glomerular basement membrane
GBMI	guilty but mentally ill
GBP	gastric bypass
GBS	gallbladder series
	gastric bypass surgery
	group B streptococci
	Guillain-Barre syndrome
GC	gas chromatography
	geriatric chair (Gerichair)
	gonococci (gonorrhea)
	good condition
	graham crackers
GCI	General Cognitive Index
G−C	Gram-negative cocci
G+C	Gram-positive cocci
GCDFP	gross cystic disease fluid protein
GCIIS	glucose control insulin infusion system
GCM	good central maintained
GCS	Glasgow Coma Scale
GCSF	granulocyte colony-stimulating factor
GCT	general care and treatment
	giant cell tumor
GCU	gonococcal urethritis
GD	Graves' disease
Gd	gadolinium
G and D	growth and development
GDF	gel diffusion precipitin
GDM	gestational diabetes mellitus
GE	gainfully employed
	gastric emptying
	gastroenteritis
	gastroesophageal
GEN/ ENDO	general anesthesia with endotracheal intubation
GENT	gentamicin
GENTA/P	gentamicin-peak
GENTA/T	gentamicin-trough
GEP	gastroenteropancreatic
GER	gastroesophageal reflux
GERD	gastroesophageal reflux disease
GET	gastric emptying time
	graded exercise test
GETA	general endotracheal anesthesia
GF	gastric fistula
	glutenfree
	grandfather
GFAP	glial fibrillary acid protein
GFD	gluten-free diet
GFM	good fetal movement
GFR	glomerular filtration rate
	grunting, flaring, and retractions
GG	gamma globulin
	guaifenesin
GGE	generalize glandular enlargement
GGS	glands, goiter, and stiffness
GGT	gamma-glutamyl transpeptidase
GGTP	gamma glutamyl transpeptidase
GH	growth hormone
GHB	gamma hydroxybutyrate
GHb	glycosylated hemoglobin
GHD	growth hormone deficiency
GHQ	General Health Questionnaire
GI	gastrointestinal
	granuloma inguinale
GIB	gastric ileal bypass
GIC	general immunocompetence
GIDA	Gastrointestinal Diagnostic Area
GIFT	gamete intrafallopian transfer

GIK	glucose-insulin-potassium
ging	gingiva
GIP	gastric inhibitory peptide
	giant cell interstitial pneumonia
GIS	gas in stomach
	gastrointestinal series
GIT	gastrointestinal tract
GITS	gastrointestinal therapeutic system
GITSG	Gastrointestinal Tumor Study Group
GIWU	gastrointestinal work-up
giv	given
GJ	gastrojejunostomy
GL	gastric lavage
	greatest length
GLA	gingivolinguoaxial
GLC	gas-liquid chromatography
GLP	Gambro Liendia Plate
GLU 5	five hour glucose tolerance test
GLYCOS Hb	glycosylated hemoglobin
GM	gram
	grand mal
	grandmother
GM +	Gram-positive
GM −	Gram-negative
gm %	grams per 100 milliliters
GMC	general medical clinic
GM-CSF	granulocyte macrophage colony stimulating factor
GMP	guanosine monophosphate
GMS	general medical services
	Gomori methenamine silver
GM&S	general medicine and surgery
GMTs	geometric mean antibody titers
GN	glomerulonephritis
	graduate nurse
	Gram negative
GNB	Gram-negative bacilli
GND	Gram-negative diplococci
GNID	Gram-negative intracellular diplococci
GNR	Gram-negative rods
GnRH	gonadotropin-releasing hormone
GOD	glucose oxidase
GOG	Gynecologic Oncology Group
GOK	God only knows
GON	gonococcal ophthalmia neonatorum
GOO	gastric outlet obstruction
GOR	general operating room
GOT	glucose oxidase test
	glutamic-oxaloacetic transaminase (aspartate aminotransferase)
	goals of treatment
GP	general practitioner
	Gram-positive
	gutta percha
G/P	gravida/para
G_4P_{3104}	four pregnancies (gravid), 3 went to term, one premature, no abortion (or miscarriage) and 4 living children (p = para)
GPC	giant papillary conjunctivitis
	Gram positive cocci
GPC/TP	glycerylphosphorylcholine to total phosphate
G6PD	glucose-6-phosphate dehydrogenase
G-PLT	giant platelets
GPMAL	gravida, para, multiple births, abortions, and live births
GPN	graduate practical nurse
GPS	Goodpasture's syndrome
GPT	glutamic pyruvic transaminase
gr	grain (approximately 60 mg) (this is a dangerous abbreviation)
G−R	Gram-negative rods
G+R	Gram-positive rods
GRASS	gradient recalled acquisition in a steady state
Grav.	gravid (pregnant)

GRD gastroesophageal reflux disease
GRE gradient-echo
GR-FR grandfather
GR-MO grandmother
GRN granules
green
$Gr_1P_0AB_1$ one pregnancy, no births, and one abortion
GRT gastric residence time
Graduate Respiratory Therapist
GRTT Graduate Respiratory Therapist Technician
GS gallstone
generalized seizure
general surgery
Gram stain
grip strength
GSD glucogen storage disease
GSD-1 glycogen storage disease, type 1
GSE genital self-examination
gluten sensitive enteropathy
grip strong and equal
GSI genuine stress incontinence
GSP general survey panel
GSPN greater superficial petrosal neurectomy
GSR galvanic skin resistance
GST gold sodium thiomalate
GSTM gold sodium thiomalate
GSW gunshot wound
GSWA gunshot wound to abdomen
GT gait
gait training
gastrotomy tube
group therapy
GTCS generalized tonic-clonic seizure
GTF gastrostomy tube feedings
GTN gestational trophoblastic neoplasms
glomerulo-tubulo-nephritis
GTP glutamyl transpeptidase
GTS Gilles de la Tourette syndrome
GTT drop
glucose tolerance test
GTT agar gelatin-tellurite-taurocholate agar
GTT3H glucose tolerence test 3 hours (oral)
GTTS drops
GU genitourinary
GUS genitourinary sphincter
genitourinary system
GVF Goldmann visual fields
good visual fields
GVHD graft-versus-host disease
G/W glucose water
GWA gunshot wound of the abdomen
GWT gunshot wound of the throat
GXP graded exercise program
GZTS Guilford-Zimmerman Temperament Survey

H

H heart
height
Hemophilis
heroin
hour
husband
hydrogen
hyperopia
hypermetropia
hypodermic
(H) hypodermic injection
H^2 hiatal hernia
H_2 hydrogen
3H high, hot, and a helluva lot
HA headache
hearing aid
hemadsorption
hemolytic anemia
hospital admission
hyperalimentation
hypermetropic astigmatism
hypothalmic amenorrhea
H/A head-to-abdomen (ratio)

HAA hepatitis-associated antigen
HACS hyperactive child syndrome
HAD human adjuvant disease
HAE hearing aid evaluation
hepatic artery embolization
hereditary angioedema
HAGG hyperimmune antivariola gamma globulin
HAI hemagglutination inhibition assay
hepatic arterial infusion
HAL hyperalimentation
HALO halothane
HAM human albumin microspheres
HAMA human anti-mouse antibody
HAM-A Hamilton Anxiety (scale)
HAM D Hamilton Depression (scale)
HAN heroin associated nephropathy
HANE hereditary angioneurotic edema
HAP hospital-acquired pneumonia
HAPC hospital-acquired penetration contact
HAPE high altitude pulmonary edema
HAPS hepatic arterial perfusion scintigraphy
HAPTO haptoglobin
HAQ Headache Assessment Questionnaire
HAR high altitude retinopathy
HARH high altitude retinal hemorrhage
HARS Hamilton Anxiety Rating Scale
HAS Hamilton Anxiety (Rating) Scale
hyperalimentation solution
HASHD hypertensive arteriosclerotic heart disease
HAT head, arms, and trunk
hospital arrival time
HAV hallux abducto valgus
hepatitis A virus
HB heart block
heel to buttock
hemoglobin (Hb)
hold breakfast
housebound
1 HB first degree heart block
HbA_{1c} glycosylated hemoglobin
HBAC hyperdynamic beta-adrenergic circulatory
HBBW hold breakfast for blood work
HB core hepatits B core antigen
HBD has been drinking
hydroxybutyric acid dehydrogenase
HB_e AB hepatitis B_e antibody
HB_e AG hepatitis B_e antigen
HBF fetal hemoglobin
hepatic blood flow
HBGM home blood glucose monitoring
HBI hemibody irradiation
HBID hereditary benign intraepithelial dyskeratosis
HBIG hepatitis B immune globulin
Hb Kansas mutant hemoglobin with a low affinity for oxygen
HBLV B-lymphotropic virus human
HBO hyperbaric oxygen
HbO_2 hyperbaric oxygen
hemoglobin, oxygenated
HBOT hyperbaric oxygen treatment
HBP high blood pressure
HBPM home blood pressure monitoring
HBS Health Behavior Scale
HbS sickle cell hemoglobin
HBεAg hepatitis B surface antigen
HbSC sickle cell hemoglobin C

HBSS	Hank's balanced salt solution
HBV	hepatitis B vaccine hepatitis B virus honey-bee venom
HBW	high birth weight
H/BW	heart-to-body weight (ratio)
HC	handicapped head circumference heel cords Hickman catheter home care housecall hydrocortisone
H & C	hot and cold
HCA	health care aide
H-CAP	hexamethylmelamine, cyclophosphamide, doxorubicin, and cisplatin
HCC	hepatocellular carcinoma
HCD	hydrocolloid dressing
HCG	human chorionic gonadotropin
HCl	hydrochloric acid hydrochloride
HCL	hairy cell leukemia
HCLs	hard contact lenses
HCM	health care maintenance hypertropic cardiomyopathy
HCMV	human cytomegalovirus infections
HCO_3	bicarbonate
HCP	hereditary coporphyria
17-HCS	17-hydroxycorticosteroids
HCT	hematocrit histamine challenge test human chorionic thyrotropin hydrochlorothiazide (this is a dangerous abbreviation) hydrocortisone
HCTU	home cervical traction unit
HCTZ	hydrochlorothiazide (this is a dangerous abbreviation)
HCVD	hypertensive cardiovascular disease
HCWs	health-care workers
HD	haloperidol decanoate hearing distance heart disease heloma durum hemodialysis high dose hip disarticulation Hodgkin's disease hospital day house dust Huntington's disease
HDAC	high-dose cytarabine
HDARAC	high dose cytarabine (ARA C)
HDCV	human diploid cell vaccine
HDL	high-density lipoprotein
HDLW	hearing distance for watch in left ear
HDMTX	high-dose methotrexate
HDMTX-CF	high-dose methotrexate and citrovorum factor
HDMTX/LV	high dose methotrexate and leucovorin
HDN	hemolytic disease of the newborn
HDP	hydroxymethyline diphosphonate
HDPAA	heparin-dependent platelet-associated antibody
HDRS	Hamilton Depression Rating Scale
HDRW	hearing distance for watch in right ear
HDS	Hamilton Depression (Rating) Scale
HDU	hemodialysis unit
HDV	hepatitis delta virus
HE	hard exudate
H&E	hematoxylin and eosin hemorrhage and exudate heredity and environment
HEAT	human erythrocyte agglutination test
HEC	Health Education Center

HEENT	head, eyes, ears, nose, and throat
HEK	human embryonic kidney
HEL	human embryonic lung
HELA	Helen Lake (tumor cells)
HELLP Syndrome	hemolysis, elevated liver enzymes, and low platelet count
HEMI	hemiplegia
HEMOSID	hemosiderin
HEMPAS	hereditary erythrocytic multinuclearity with positive acidified serum test
HEMS	helicopter emergency medical services
HEP	heparin
	hepatic
	histamine equivalent prick
HEPA	hamster egg penetration assay
hep cap	heparin cap
HERP	human exposure (dose)/rodent potency (dose)
HES	hydroxyethyl starch
	hypereosinophilic syndrome
Hex	hexamethylmelamine
Hexa-CAF	hexamethylmelamine, cyclophosphamide, methotrexate, and fluorouracil
HF	hard feces
	hay fever
	head of fetus
	heart failure
	high frequency
	house formula
HFA	health facility administrator
HFD	high fiber diet
	high forceps delivery
HFHL	high-frequence hearing loss
HFI	hereditary fructose intolerance
HFJV	high frequency jet ventilation
H flu	Hemophilus influenzae
HFPPV	high-frequency positive pressure ventilation
HFST	hearing-for-speech test
HFUPR	hourly fetal urine production rate
HFV	high-frequency ventilation
HG	hemoglobin
Hgb	hemoglobin
HGH	human growth hormone
HGO	hip guidance orthosis
HGPRT	hypoxanthine-guanine phosphoribosyl-transferase
HH	hard of hearing
	hiatal hernia
	home health
	hypogonadotrophic hypogonadism
H&H	hematocrit and hemoglobin
HHA	hereditary hemolytic anemia
	home health agency
HHC	home health care
HHD	home hemodialysis
	hypertensive heart disease
HHFM	high humidity face mask
HHM	humoral hypercalcemia of malignancy
HHN	hand held nebulizer
HHNC	hyperosmolar hyperglycemic nonketotic coma
HHNK	hyperglycemic hyperosmolar nonketotic (coma)
HHS	Health and Human Service (US Department of)
HHT	hereditary hemorrhagic telangiectasis
HHTC	high-humidity trach collar
HHTM	high-humidity trach mask
HI	head injury
	hearing impaired
	hemagglutination inhibition
	hospital insurance
HIA	hemagglutination inhibition antibody

5-HIAA 5 hydroxyindoleacetic acid
HIB Haemophilus influenzae type b (vaccine)
hi-cal high caloric
HID headache, insomnia, and depression
herniated intervertebral disc
HIDA hepato-iminodiacetic acid (lidofenin)
HIE hypoxic-ischemic encephalopathy
HIF *haemophilus influenzae*
higher integrative functions
HIHA high impulsiveness, high anxiety
HIL hypoxic-ischemic lesion
HILA high impulsiveness, low anxiety
HIR head injury routine
HIS Hanover Intensive Score
Health Intention Scale
hospital information system
HISMS How I See Myself Scale
Histo histoplasmin skin test
HIT heparin induced thrombocytopenia
histamine inhalation test
HIU head injury unit
HIV human immunodeficiency virus
HIVD herniated intervertebral disc
HJB Howell-Jolly bodies
HJR hepato-jugular reflex
H-K hand to knee
HKAFO hip-knee-ankle-foot orthosis
HKAO hip-knee-ankle orthosis
HKO hip-knee orthosis
HKS heel, knee, and shin
HL hairline
half-life
hallux limitus
haloperidol
harelip
hearing level
heparin lock
Hickman line
H&L heart and lung
HLA negative heart, lungs, and abdomen negative
HLA human lymphocyte antigen
HLD haloperidol decanoate
herniated lumbar disc
HLHS hypoplastic left heart syndrome
HLK heart, liver, and kidney
HLT heart-lung transplantation
HLV herpes-like virus
hypoplastic left ventricle
HM hand motion
heart murmur
heavily muscled
hemola molle
Holter monitor
human milk
human semisynthetic insulin
HMA hemorrhages and microaneurysms
HMB homatropine methylbromide
HMBA hexamethylene bisacetamide
HMD hyaline membrane disease
HME heat, massage, and exercise
HMDP hydroxymethyline diphosphonate
HMETSC heavy metal screen
HMG human menopausal gonadotropin
HMG CoA hepatic hydroxymethyl glutaryl coenzyme A
HMI healed myocardial infarction
HMK homemaking
HMM hexamethylmelamine
HMO Health Maintenance Organization
HMP hexose monophosphate
hot moist packs
HMPAO hexamethylpropylenamine oxide

HMR	histocytic medullary reticulosis
HMX	heat massage exercise
HN	head and neck
	head nurse
	high nitrogen
H&N	head and neck
HNC	hyperosmolar nonketotic coma
HN_2	mechlorethamine HCl
HNKDC	hyperosomolar nonketotic diabetic coma
HNKDS	hyperosmolar nonketotic diabetic state
HNLN	hospitalization no longer necessary
HNP	herniated nucleus pulposus
HNRNA	heterogeneous nuclear ribonucleic acid
HNS	head and neck surgery
	head, neck, and shaft
HNV	has not voided
HO	hand orthosis
	Hemotology-Oncology
	heterotropic ossification
	hip orthosis
	house officer
H/O	history of
H_2O	water
H_2O_2	hydrogen peroxide
HOA	hip osteoarthritis
HOB	head of bed
HOB UPSOB	head of bed up for shortness of breath
HOC	Health Officer Certificate
HOCM	high osmolar contrast media
	hypertrophic obstructive cardiomyopathy
HOG	halothane, oxygen, and gas (nitrous oxide)
HOH	hard of hearing
HOI	hospital onset of infection
HOM	high osmolar contrast media
HONDA	hypertensive, obese, Negro, diabetic, arthritic
HOPI	history of present illness
HP	hard palate
	hemipelvectomy
	hemiplegia
	hot packs
	hydrogen peroxide
	hydrophilic petrolatum
H&P	history and physical
HPA	hypothalamic-pituitary-adrenal (axis)
HPE	history and physical examination
HPF	high-power field
HPFH	hereditary persistence of fetal hemoglobin
HPI	history of present illness
HPL	human placenta lactogen
HPLC	high-pressure (performance) liquid chromatography
HPG	human pituitary gonadotropin
HPL	hyperplexia
HPM	hemiplegic migraine
HPN	home parenteral nutrition
HPO	hydrophilic ointment
	hypertrophic pulmonary osteoarthropathy
HPS	hypertrophic pyloric stenosis
HPT	histamine provocation test
	hyperparathyroidism
hPTH	human parathyroid hormone I_{34} (teriparatide)
HPTM	home prothrombin time monitoring
HPV	human papilloma virus
	human parvovirus
HPZ	high pressure zone
HQC	hydroquinone cream
HR	hallux rigidus
	Harrington rod
	heart rate
	hospital record
	hour
H & R	hysterectomy and radiation
HRA	high right atrium
	histamine releasing activity

HRC	Human Rights Committee
HRCT	high-resolution computer tomography
HRF	Harris return flow
	histamine releasing factor
HRIF	histamine inhibitory releasing factor
HRL	head rotated left
HRLA	human reovirus-like agent
HRP	high-risk pregnancy
	horseradish peroxidase
HRR	head rotated right
HRS	hepatorenal syndrome
HRT	heart rate
	hormone replacement therapy
HS	bedtime
	half strength
	hamstrings
	Hartman's solution (lactated Ringer's)
	heart sounds
	heavy smoker
	heel spur
	heel stick
	hereditary spherocytosis
	herpes simplex
	high school
H→S	heel to shin
H&S	hemorrhage and shock
	hysterectomy and sterilization
HSA	Health Systems Agency
	human serum albumin
	hypersomnia-sleep apnea
HSBG	heel stick blood gas
HSCL	Hopkins Symptom Check List
HSE	herpes simplex encephalitis
HSG	herpes simplex genitalis
	histosalpingogram
HSL	herpes simplex labialis
HSM	hepato-splenomegaly
	holosystolic murmur
HSP	Henoch-Schonlein purpura
	hysterosalpingography
HSR	heated serum reagin
HSSE	high soap suds enema
	histotechnologist
HSV	herpes simplex virus
HSVI	herpes simplex virus type 1
HT	hammertoe
	hearing test
	heart
	heart transplant
	height
	high temperature
	hyperthermia
	hubbard tank
	hypermetropia
	hyperopia
	hypertension
H&T	hospitalization and treatment
H(T)	intermittent hypertropia
5-HT	5-hydroxytryptamine
ht. aer.	heated aerosol
HTAT	human tetanus antitoxin
HTB	hot tub bath
HTC	hypertensive crisis
HTF	house tube feeding
HTK	heel to knee
HTL	hearing threshold level
	human T-cell leukemia
	human thymic leukemia
HTLV III	human T cell lymphotrophic virus type III
HTN	hypertension
HTP	House-Tree-Person-test
5-HTP	5-hydroxytryptophan
HTS	head traumatic syndrome
	heel-to-shin
HTT	hand thrust test
HTV	herpes-type virus
HTVD	hypertensive vascular disease
HU	head unit
	hydroxyurea
HUIFM	human leukocyte interferon meloy
HUK	human urinary kallikrein
HUR	hydroxyurea
HUS	hemolytic uremic syndrome
	husband

husb husband
HV hallux valgus
 has voided
 Hemovac®
 home visit
H&V hemigastrecotomy and vagotomy
HVA homovanillic acid
HVGS high volt galvanic stimulation
HVL half value layer
HW heparin well
 housewife
hwb hot water bottle
HWFE housewife
HWP hot wet pack
Hx history
 hospitalization
HXM hexamethylmelamine
Hy hypermetropia
HYG hygiene
Hyper Al hyperalimentation
hypopit hypopituitarism
Hyst hysterectomy
Hz Hertz
HZ herpes zoster
HZO herpes zoster ophthalmicus
HZV herpes zoster virus

I

I impression
 incisal
 independent
 initial
 inspiration
 intact (bag of waters)
 intermediate
 one
I_2 iodine
I^{131} radioactive iodine
IA incidental appendectomy
 intra-amniotic
I & A irrigation and aspiration
IAA interrupted aortic arch
IABC intra-aortic balloon counterpulsation
IABP intra-aortic balloon pump
IAC internal auditory canal
 intra-arterial chemotherapy
IAC-CPR interposed abdominal compressions—cardio-pulmonary resuscitation
IACP intra-aortic counterpulsation
IADHS inappropriate antidiuretic hormone syndrome
IA DSA intra-arterial subtraction arteriography
IAGT indirect antiglobulin test
IAHA immune adherence hemagglutination
IAI intra-abdominal infection
IAM internal auditory meatus
IAN intern admission note
IAO immediately after onset
IAP intermittent acute porphyria
IASD interatrial septal defect
 immunoaugmentive therapy
IAT indirect antiglobulin test
IAV intermittent assist ventilation
IB ileal bypass
 isolation bed
IBBB intra-blood-brain barrier
IBBBB incomplete bilateral bundle branch block
IBC iron binding capacity
IBD inflammatory bowel disease
IBI intermittent bladder irrigation
ibid at the same place
IBILI indirect bilirubin
IBNR incurred but not reported
IBOW intact bag of waters
IBRS Inpatient Behavior Rating Scale
IBS irritable bowel syndrome
IBU ibuprofen
IBW ideal body weight
IC between meals
 immunocompromised
 incomplete
 indirect Coombs (test)

	individual counseling
	inspiratory capacity
	intensive care
	intercostal
	intermediate care
	intermittent catheterization
	interstitial changes
	intracranial
	irritable colon
ICA	intermediate care area
	internal carotid artery
	islet-cell antibody
ICB	intracranial bleeding
ICBT	intercostobronchial trunk
ICC	islet cell carcinoma
ICCE	intracapsular cataract extraction
ICCU	intensive coronary care unit
	intermediate coronary care unit
ICD	instantaneous cardiac death
	isocitrate dehydrogenase
ICD 9 CM	International Classification of Diseases, 9th Revision, Clinical Modification
ICDC	implantable cardioverter-defibrillator catheter
ICDO	international classification of diseases for oncology
ICE	ice, compression, and elevation
	individual career exploration
ICF	intermediate care facility
	intracellular fluid
ICG	indocyanine green
ICH	immunocompromised host
	intracerebral hemorrhage
	intracranial hemorrhage
ICL	intracorneal lense
ICM	intracostal margin
ICN	infection control nurse
	intensive care nursery
ICP	intracranial pressure
ICPP	intubated continuous positive pressure
ICRF-159	razoxane
ICS	ileocecal sphincter
	intercostal space
ICSH	interstitial cell-stimulating hormone
ICT	icterus
	indirect Coombs' test
	inflammation of connective tissue
	intensive conventional therapy
	intermittent cervical traction
	intracranial tumor
ICU	intensive care unit
	intermediate care unit
ICV	intracerebroventricular
ICVH	ischemic cerebrovascular headache
ICW	intercellular water
ID	identification
	identify
	ifosfamide, mesna uroprotection, and doxorubicin
	immunodiffusion
	infectious disease (physician or department)
	initial diagnosis
	initial dose
	injected dose
	intradermal
id	the same
I & D	incision and drainage
IDA	iron deficiency anemia
IDDM	insulin-dependent diabetes mellitus
IDDS	implantable drug delivery system
IDE	Investigational Device Exemption
IDFC	immature dead female child
IDG	interdisciplinary group
IDI	Interpersonal Dependency Inventory

IDK internal derangement of knee
IDM infant of a diabetic mother
IDMC immature dead male child
IDR intradermal reaction
IDS infectious disease service
IDU idoxuridine
IDV intermittent demand ventilation
IDVC indwelling venous catheter
IE immunoelectrophoresis
induced emesis
inner ear
international unit (European abbreviation)
i.e. that is
I:E ratio inspiratory to expiratory time ratio
I&E internal and external
IEC inpatient exercise center
IEF iso-electric focusing
IEM immune electron microscopy
IEP immunoelectrophoresis
individualized education program
IF ifosfamide
immunofluorescence
interferon
intermaxillary fixation
internal fixation
intrinsic factor
involved field (radiotherapy)
IFA indirect fluorescent antibody immunofluorescent assay
IFE immunofixation electrophoresis
IFM internal fetal monitoring
IFN interferon
IFOS ifosfamide
IFP inflammatory fibroid polyps
IgA immunoglobulin A
IgD immunoglobulin D
IGDE idiopathic gait disorders of the elderly
IGDM infant of gestational diabetic mother
IgE immunoglobulin E
IgG immunoglobulin G
IGIM immune globulin intramuscular
IGIV immune globulin intravenous
IgM immunoglobulin M
IGR intrauterine growth retardation
IGT impaired glucose tolerance
IH indirect hemagglutination
infectious hepatitis
inguinal hernia
IHA immune hemolytic anemia
indirect hemagglutination
IHC immobilization hypercalcemia
IHD intraheptic duct (ule)
ischemic heart disease
IHH idiopathic hypogona-dotrophic hypogo nadism
IHS Indian Health Service
Iodiopathic Headache Score
IHs iris hamartomas
IHSA iodinated human serum albumin
IHSS idiopathic hypertrophic subaortic stenosis
IHT insulin hypoglycemia test
IHW inner heel wedge
IIA internal iliac artery
IICP increased intracranial pressure
IICU infant intensive care unit
IJ ileojejunal
internal jugular
IJD inflammatory joint disease
IJR idiojunctional rhythm
IJT idiojunctional tachycardia
IJV internal jugular vein
IK immobilized knee
interstitial keratitis

IL	immature lungs interleukin (1, 2, and 3) Intralipid®
ILA	indicated low forceps
ILBBB	incomplete left bundle branch block
ILBW	infant, low birth weight
ILD	interstitial lung disease ischemic leg disease
ILE	infantile lobar emphysema
ILFC	immature living female child
ILM	internal limiting membrane
ILMC	immature living male child
ILMI	inferolateral myocardial infarct
ILVEN	inflammatory linear verrucal epidermal nevus
IM	infectious mononucleosis intermetatarsal internal medicine intramuscular
IMA	inferior mesenteric artery internal mammary artery
IMAC	ifosfamide, mesna uroprotection, doxorubicin, and cisplatin
IMAG	internal mammary artery graft
IMB	intermenstrual bleeding
IMC	intramedullary catheter
IMCU	intermediate care unit
IME	independent medical examination
IMF	ifosfamide, mesna uroprotection, methotrexate, and fluorouracil intermaxillary fixation
IMG	internal medicine group (group practices)
IMH test	indirect microhemagglutination test
IMI	imipramine inferior myocardial infarction
IMIG	intramuscular immunoglobulin
IMLC	incomplete mitral leaflet closure
IMN	internal mammary (lymph) node
IMP	impacted important impression improved
IMS	incurred in military service
IMT	inspiratory muscle training
IMV	inferior mesenteric vein intermittent mandatory ventilation
IMVP-16	ifosfamide, mesna uroprotection, methotrexate, and etoposide
In	inches indium
INC	incisal incision incomplete incontinent increase inside-the-needle catheter
Inc Spir	incentive spirometer
IND	induced Investigational New Drug (application)
INDM	infant of nondiabetic mother
INEX	inexperienced
INF	infant infarction infected inferior information infused infusion
INFC	infected infection
ING	inguinal
✓ ing	checking
INH	isoniazid
inj	injection injury

INK	injury not known
INO	internuclear ophthalmoplegia
INDO	indomethacin
inpt	inpatient
INS	insurance
INST	instrumental delivery
INT	intermittent needle therapy
	internal
Int mon	internal monitor
INTERP	interpretation
intol	intolerance
int-rot	internal rotation
int trx	intermittent traction
intub	intubation
inver	inversion
I&O	intake and output
IO	inferior oblique
	initial opening
	intraocular pressure
IOC	intern on call
	intraoperative cholangiogram
IOCG	intraoperative cholangiogram
IOD	interorbital distance
IODM	infant of diabetic mother
IOF	intraocular fluid
IOFB	intraocular foreign body
IOH	idiopathic orthostatic hypotension
IOI	intraosseous infusion
IOL	intraocular lens
ION	ischemic optic neuropathy
IOP	intraocular pressure
IORT	intraoperative radiation therapy
IOS	intraoperative sonography
IOV	initial office visit
IP	incubation period
	individualized plan
	interphalangeal
	intraperitoneal
IPA	invasive pulmonary aspergillosis
	isopropyl alcohol
IPCD	infantile polycystic disease
IPD	immediate pigment darkening
	inflammatory pelvic disease
	intermittent peritoneal dialysis
	interpupillary distance
IPF	idiopathic pulmonary fibrosis
IPFD	intrapartum fetal distress
IPG	impedance plethysmography
	individually polymerized grass
IPH	interphalangeal
IPJ	interphalangeal joint
IPK	intractable plantar keratosis
IPMI	inferoposterior myocardial infarct
IPN	infantile periarteritis nodosa
	intern's progress note
IPOF	immediate postoperative fitting
IPOP	immediate postoperative prosthesis
IPP	inflatable penile prosthesis
IPPA	inspection, palpation, percussion, and auscultation
IPPB	intermittent positive pressure breathing
IPPI	interruption of pregnancy for psychiatric indication
IPPV	intermittent positive pressure ventilation
IPS	infundibular pulmonic stenosis
IPSF	immediate postsurgical fitting
IPV	inactivated polio vaccine
IPVC	interpolated premature ventricular contraction
IPW	interphalangeal width
IQ	intelligence quotient
IR	inferior rectus
	infrared

	internal rotation
I&R	insertion and removal
IRA-EEA	ileorectal anastomoses with end-to-end anastomosis
IRB	institutional review board
IRBBB	incomplete right bundle branch block
IRBC	immature red blood cell
IRBP	interphotoreceptor retinoid-binding protein
IRC	indirect radionuclide cystography
IRCU	intensive respiratory care unit
IRDS	idiopathic respiratory distress syndrome
	infant respiratory distress syndrome
IRH	intraretinal hemorrhage
IRMA	immunoradiometric assay
	intraretinal microvascular abnormalities
IROS	ipsilateral routing of signals
IRR	intrarenal reflux
irreg	irregular
IRT	immunoreactive trypsin
IRV	inspiratory reserve volume
IS	incentive spirometer
	induced sputum
	intercostal space
	inventory of systems
	ipecac syrup
I/S	instruct/supervise
ISB	incentive spirometry breathing
ISC	isolette servo control
ISCs	irreversible sickle cells
ISD	inhibited sexual desire
	initial sleep disturbance
ISDN	isosorbide dinitrate
ISG	immune serum globulin
ISH	isolated systolic hypertension
ISMA	infantile spinal muscular atrophy
ISO	isoproterenol
ISQ	as before; continue on (*in status quo*)
ISS	Injury Severity Score
IS10S	10% invert sugar in saline
IST	insulin sensitivity test
	insulin shock therapy
ISW	interstitial water
IS10W	10% invert sugar in water
ISWI	incisional surgical wound infection
IT	inferior-temporal
	inhalation therapy
	intensive therapy
	intermittent traction
	intertuberous
	intrathecal
ITA	individual treatment assessment
ITAG	internal thoracic artery graft
ITB	iliotibial band
ITC	Incontinence Treatment Center
ITCP	idiopathic thrombocytopenia purpura
ITCU	intensive thoracic cardiovascular unit
ITE	insufficient therapeutic effect
	in-the-ear (hearing aid)
ITGV	intrathoracic gas volume
ITP	idiopathic thrombocytopenic purpura
	interim treatment plan
ITT	identical twins (raised) together
	insulin tolerance test
ITVAD	indwelling transcutaneous vascular access device
IU	international unit (this is a dangerous abbreviation as it is read as intravenous)
IUC	intrauterine catheter
IUD	intrauterine death
	intrauterine device
IUDR	idoxuridine
IUFD	intrauterine fetal death
	intrauterine fetal distress

IUGR intrauterine growth retardation
IUI intrauterine insemination
IUP intrauterine pregnancy
IUPC intrauterine pressure catheter
IUPD intrauterine pregnancy delivered
IUP,TBCS intrauterine pregnancy, term birth, cesarean section
IUP,TBLC intrauterine pregnancy, term birth, living child
IUR intrauterine retardation
IV four
intravenous (i.v.)
symbol for class 4 controlled substances
IVA Intervir-A
IVAP implantable vascular access device
IVC inferior vena cava
inspiratory vital capacity
intravenous cholangiogram
intraventricular catheter
IVCD intraventricular conduction defect
IVD intervertebral disk
intravenous drip
IVDA intravenous drug abuse
IVF *in vitro* fertilization
intravenous fluid(s)
IVFE intravenous fat emulsion
IVF-ET *in vitro* fertilization-embryo transfer
IVFT intravenous fetal transfusion
IVGTT intravenous glucose tolerance test
IVH intravenous hyperalimentation
intraventricular hemorrhage
IVIG intravenous immunoglobulin
IVJC intervertebral joint complex
IVL intravenous lock
IVLBW infant of very low birth weight
IVOX intravascular oxygenator
IVP intravenous push
intravenous pyelogram
IVPB intravenous piggyback
IVPU intravenous push
IVR idioventricular rhythm
IVS intraventricular septum
irritable voiding syndrome
IVSD intraventricular septal defect
IVSE interventricular septal excursion
IVSS intravenous Soluset®
IVTTT intravenous tolbutamide tolerance test
IVU intravenous urography
IWL insensible water loss
IWMI inferior wall myocardial infarct
IWML idiopathic white matter lesion
IWT impacted wisdom teeth

J

J Jewish
joint
juice
JAMG juvenile autoimmune myasthenia gravis
JBE Japanese B encephalitis
JC junior clinicians (medical students)
JD jaundice
JDMS juvenile dermatomyositis
JE Japanese encephalitis
JER junctional escape rhythm
JF joint fluid
JFS Jewish Family Service
JHR Jarisch-Herxheimer reaction
JI jejunoileal
JIB jejunoileal bypass
JIS juvenile idiopathic scoliosis
JJ jaw jerk

JLP	juvenile laryngeal papillomatosis
JM-9	iproplatin
JMS	junior medical student
JND	just noticeable difference
jnt	joint
JODM	juvenile onset diabetes mellitus
JOMAC	judgment, orientation, memory, affect, and cognition
JOMACI	judgment, orientation, memory, abstraction, and calculation intact
JP	Jackson-Pratt (drain)
	Jobst pump
	joint protection
JPB	junctional premature beats
JPC	junctional premature contraction
JPS	joint position sense
JPTS	juvenile tropical pancreatitis syndrome
JRA	juvenile rheumatoid arthritis
JRAN	junior resident admission note
Jr BF	junior baby food
JRC	joint replacement center
JT	jejunostomy tube
	joint
JTF	jejunostomy tube feeding
JTP	joint projection
J-Tube	jejunostomy tube
juv.	juvenile
JVD	jugular venous distention
JVP	jugular venous pressure
	jugular venous pulse
JVPT	jugular venous pulse tracing
JW	Jehovah's witness
JXG	juvenile xanthogranuloma

K

K	potassium
	thousand
	vitamin K
K_1	phytonadione
K_3	menadione
K_4	menadiol sodium diphosphate
17K	17-ketosteroids
KA	ketoacidosis
KAB	knowledge, attitude, and behavior
KABINS	knowledge, attitude, behavior, and improvement in nutritional status
KAFO	knee-ankle-foot orthosis
KAO	knee-ankle orthosis
KAS	Katz Adjustment Scale
KASH	knowledge, abilities, skills, and habits
K-A units	King-Armstrong units
KC	keratoconjunctivitis
	knees to chest
kcal	kilocalorie
kCi	kilocurie
KCl	potassium chloride
KCS	keratoconjunctivitis sicca
KD	Kawasaki's disease
	Keto Diastex®
	kidney donors
	knee disarticulation
KDA	known drug allergies
17 Keto	17 ketosteroids
KF	kidney function
KFAO	knee-foot-ankle orthosis
KFD	Kyasanur Forrest disease
KFR	Kayser-Fleischer ring
kg	kilogram
KGC	Keflin®, gentamicin, and carbenicillin
K24H	potassium, urine 24 hour
KI	karyopyknotic index
	knee immobilizer
	potassium iodide
KID	keratitis, ichthyosis, and deafness (syndrome)
kilo	kilogram
KISS	saturated solution of potassium iodide
KIT	Kahn intelligence test
KJ	kilojoule
	knee jerk
KK	knee kick
KL-BET	Kleihauer-Betke

Kleb	Klebsiella
KLH	keyhole limpet hemocyanin
KLS	kidneys, liver, and spleen
KM	kanamycin
$KMnO_4$	potassium permanganate
KNO	keep needle open
KO	keep open
	knee orthosis
KOH	potassium hydroxide
KP	hot pack
	keratoprecipitate
Kr	krypton
KS	Kaposi's sarcoma
17-KS	17-ketosteroids
KSA	knowledge, skills, and abilities
KS/OI	Kaposi's sarcoma and opportunistic infections
KT	kidney transplant
KTU	kidney transplant unit
KUB	kidney, ureter, and bladder
KUS	kidney(s), ureter(s), and spleen
KV	kilovolt
KVO	keep vein open
KVP	kilovolt peak
KW	Keith-Wagener (ophthalmoscopic finding, graded I-IV)
	Kimmelstiel-Wilson
KWB	Keith, Wagener, Barker
K-wire	Kirschner wire

L

L	fifty
	left
	lente insulin
	lingual
	liter
	liver
	lumbar
	lung
(L)	left
$L_1 \ldots L_5$	lumbar nerve 1 through 5
	lumbar vertebra 1 through 5
LA	language age
	Latin American
	left arm
	left atrial
	left atrium
	local anesthesia
	long acting
L + A	light and accommodation
	living and active
Lab	laboratory
LAC	laceration
	long arm cast
LACT-ART	lactate arterial
LAD	left anterior descending
	left axis deviation
LADCA	left anterior descending coronary artery
LADD	left anterior descending diagonal
LAD-MIN	left axis deviation minimal
LAE	left atrial enlargement
	long above elbow
LAF	laminar air flow
	Latin-American female
	low animal fat
	lymphocyte-activating factor
LAG	lymphangiogram
LAH	left anterior hemiblock
	left atrial hypertrophy
LAHB	left anterior hemiblock
LAK	lymphokine-activated killer
LAL	left axillary line
	limulus amebocyte lysate
LAM	laminectomy
	Latin-American male
LANC	long arm navicular cast
LAN	lymphadenopathy
LAO	left anterior oblique
LAP	laparoscopy
	laparotomy
	left arterial pressure
	leucine amino peptidase
	leukocyte alkaline phosphatase
LAPMS	long arm posterior molded splint

LAPW left atrial posterior wall
LAQ long arc quad
LAR left arm, reclining
LAS laxative abuse syndrome
leucine acetylsalicylate
long arm splint
lymphadenopathy syndrome
lymphangioscintigraphy
L-ASP asparaginase
LAT lateral
left anterior thigh
lat.men. lateral meniscectomy
LATS long-acting thyroid stimulator
LAV lymphadenopathy associated virus
LAW left atrial wall
LB large bowel
left breast
left buttock
live births
low back
lung biopsy
pound
L&B left and below
LBB left breast biopsy
LBBB left bundle branch block
LBCD left border of cardiac dullness
LBD large bile duct
left border dullness
LBE long below elbow
LBH length, breadth, and height
LBM lean body mass
loose bowel movement
LBO large bowel obstruction
LBP low back pain
low blood pressure
LBT low back tenderness
low back trouble
LBV left brachial vein
LBW lean body weight
low birth weight
LC leisure counseling
living children
low calorie
lung cancer
LCA Leber's congenital amaurosis
left coronary artery
left circumflex artery
light contact assist
LCAT lecithin cholesterol acyltransferase
LCB left costal border
LCCA left common carotid artery
leukocytoclastic angiitis
LCCS low cervical cesarean section
LCD coal tar solution (*liquor carbonis detergens*)
localized collagen dystrophy
low calcium diet
LCF left circumflex
LCFA long-chain fatty acid
LCFM left circumflex marginal
LCGU local cerebral glucose utilization
LCH local city hospital
LCLC large cell lung carcinoma
LCM left costal margin
lymphocytic choriomeningitis
LCR late cortical response
late cutaneous reaction
LCS low constant suction
low continuous suction
LCSW Licensed Clinical Social Worker
LCT long chain triglyceride
low cervical transverse
lymphocytotoxicity
LCTD low-calcium test diet
LCV leucovorin
low cervical vertical
LCX left circumflex coronary artery
LD labor and delivery
lactic dehydrogenase (formerly LDH)
last dose
learning disability
learning disorder
Legionnaire's disease
lethal dose

	levodopa
	liver disease
	living donor
	loading dose
	longdwell
LDB	Legionnaires disease bacterium
LDDS	local dentist
LDH	lactic dehydrogenase
LDIH	left direct inguinal hernia
LDL	low-density lipoprotein
L-dopa	levodopa
LDR	labor, delivery, and recovery
LDR/P	labor, delivery, recovery, and postpartum
LDT	left dorsotransverse
LDUB	long double upright brace
LDV	laser Doppler velocimetry
LE	left ear
	left eye
	lens extraction
	live embryo
	lower extremities
	lupus erythematosus
LEA	lumbar epidural anesthesia
LED	lupus erythematosus disseminatus
LEHPZ	lower esophageal high pressure zone
LEJ	ligation of the esophagogastric junction
LEM	lateral eye movements
	light electron microscope
LEP	lower esophageal pressure
LEP 2	leptospirosis 2
LE prep	lupus erythematosus preparation
L-ERX	leukoerythroblastic reaction
LES	local excitatory state
	lower esophageal sphincter
	lupus erythematosis systemic
LESP	lower esophageal sphincter pressure
LET	linear energy transfer
LEV	levator muscle
LF	Lassa fever
	left foot
	low fat
	low forceps
	low frequency
LFA	left femoral artery
	left forearm
	left fronto-anterior
	low friction arthroplasty
LFC	living female child
	low fat and cholesterol
LFD	lactose free diet
	low fat diet
	low fiber diet
	low forceps delivery
LFL	left frontolateral
LFP	left frontoposterior
LFS	liver function series
LFT	latex flocculation test
	left frontotransverse
	liver function tests
LFU	limit flocculation unit
LG	large
	laryngectomy
	left gluteal
LGA	large for gestational age
	left gastric artery
LGI	lower gastrointestinal (series)
LGL	Lown-Ganong-Levine (syndrome)
LGN	lobular glomerulonephritis
LGV	lymphagranuloma venerum
LH	left hand
	left hyperphoria
	luteinizing hormone
LHA	left hepatic artery
LHF	left heart failure
LHG	left hand grip
LHH	left homonymous hemianopsia
LHL	left hemisphere lesions
LHP	left hemiparesis
LHR	leukocyte histamine release
LHRH	luteinizing hormone-releasing hormone (hypothalamic)

LHS	left hand side
LHT	left hypertropia
LI	lactose intolerance
	large intestine
	learning impaired
Li	lithium
LIB	left in bottle
LIC	left iliac crest
	left internal carotid
	leisure interest class
LICA	left internal carotid artery
LICD	lower intestinal Crohn's disease
LICM	left intercostal margin
Li_2CO_3	lithium carbonate
LICS	left intercostal space
Lido	lidocaine
LIF	left iliac fossa
	liver (migration) inhibitory factor
	left index finger
LIG	ligament
LIH	left inguinal hernia
LIHA	low impulsiveness, high anxiety
LILA	low impulsiveness, low anxiety
LIMA	left internal mammary artery (graft)
LING	lingual
LIO	left inferior oblique
LIP	lithium-induced polydipsia
	lymphocytic interstitial pneumonia
LIQ	liquid
	lower inner quadrant
LIR	left iliac region
	left inferior rectus
LIS	left intercostal space
	low intermittent suction
LISS	low ionic strength saline
LIV	left innominate vein
LIVC	left inferior vena cava
LIVPRO	liver profile
LJM	limited joint mobility
LK	lamellar keratoplasty
	left kidney
LKA	Lazare-Klerman-Armour (Personality Inventory)
LKKS	liver, kidneys, spleen
LKS	liver, kidneys, spleen
LKSB	liver, kidneys, spleen, and bladder
L╲ ╱M K─O S╱ ╲T	liver, kidneys, and spleen negative, no masses, or tenderness
LL	large lymphocyte
	left leg
	left lower
	left lung
	lower lid
	lower lip
	lower lobe
	lumbar length
	lymphocytic leukemia
	lymphoblastic lymphoma
LL2	limb lead two
LLA	limulus lysate assay
LLB	left lateral border
	long leg brace
LLC	long leg cast
LLBCD	left lower border of cardiac dullness
LLD	left lateral decubitus
	left length discrepancy
LLE	left lower extremity
LL-GXT	low-level graded exercise test
LLL	left lower lid
	left lower lobe (lung)
LLLE	lower lid left eye
LLLNR	left lower lobe, no rales
LLO	Lengionella-like organism
LLOD	lower lid, right eye
LLOS	lower lid, left eye
LLQ	left lower quadrant (abdomen)
LLR	left lateral rectus
LLRE	lower lid, right eye
LLS	lazy leukocyte syndrome
LLSB	left lower sternal border
LLT	left lateral thigh
LLWC	long leg walking cast
LLX	left lower extremity
L/M	liters per minute
LMA	left mento-anterior
	liver membrane autoantibody

LMB	Laurence-Moon-Biedl syndrome
LMC	living male child
LMCA	left main coronary artery
	left middle cerebral artery
LMCAT	left middle cerebral artery thrombosis
LMCL	left midclavicular line
LMD	local medical doctor
	low molecular weight dextran
LME	left mediolateral episiotomy
LMEE	left middle ear exploration
LMF	left middle finger
L/min	liters per minute
LML	left medial lateral
	left middle lobe
LMLE	left mediolateral episiotomy
LMM	lentigo maligna melanoma
LMP	last menstrual period
	left mentotposterior
LMR	left medial rectus
LMS	lateral medullary syndrome
LMT	left main trunk
	left mentotransverse
LMWD	low molecular weight dextran
LMWH	low molecular weight heparin
LN_2	liquid nitrogen
	lymph nodes
LNCs	lymph node cells
LND	light-near dissociation
	lymph node dissection
LNMP	last normal menstrual period
LO	lateral oblique (x-ray view)
	lumber orthosis
LOA	leave of absence
	left occiput anterior
	lysis of adhesions
LOC	laxative of choice
	level of care
	level of consciousness
	local
	loss of consciousness
LOCM	low-osmolar contrast media
LOD	line of duty
LOIH	left oblique inguinal hernia
LOL	left occipitolateral
	little old lady
LOM	left otitis media
	limitation of motion
	loss of motion
	low-osmolar (contrast) media
LOMSA	left otitis media, suppurative, acute
LOMSC	left otitis media, suppurative, chronic
LoNa	low sodium
LOP	leave on pass
	left occiput posterior
LOQ	lower outer quadrant
LORS-I	Level of Rehabilitation Scale-I
LOS	length of stay
LOT	left occiput transverse
	Licensed Occupational Therapist
LOV	loss of vision
LOZ	lozenge
LP	light perception
	low protein
	lumbar puncture
L/P	lactate-pyruvate ratio
LPA	left pulmonary artery
L-PAM	melphalan
LPC	laser photocoagulation
LPc̄P	light perception with projection
LPD	low protein diet
	luteal phase defect
lpf	low-power field
LPF	liver plasma flow
LPH	left posterior hemiblock
LPI	laser peripheral iridectomy
LPL	lipoprotein lipase
LPM	liters per minute
LPN	Licensed Practical Nurse
LPO	left posterior oblique
	light perception only

LPS lipopolysaccharide
LR labor room
lactated Ringer's (injection)
lateral rectus
left-right
light reflex
L→R left to right
LR1A labor room 1A
LRD living related donor
living renal donor
LREH low renin essential hypertension
LRF left rectus femoris
LRM left radical mastectomy
LRMP last regular menstrual period
LRND left radical neck dissection
LRQ lower right quadrant
LRS lactated Ringer's solution
LRT lower respiratory tract
LRTI lower respiratory tract infection
LRZ lorazepam
LS left side
legally separated
liver scan
liver-spleen
low salt
lumbosacral
L/S lecithin-spingomyelin ratio
L5-S1 lumbar fifth vertebra to sacral first vertebra
LSA left sacrum anterior
lipid-bound sialic acid
lymphosarcoma
LSB left sternal border
LS BPS laparoscopic bilateral partial salpingectomy
LSC late systolic click
LSCA left scapuloanterior
LSCP left scapuloposterior
LSD low salt diet
lysergide
LSE local side effects
LSF low saturated fat
LSKM liver-spleen-kidney-megalia
LSL left sacrolateral
left short leg (brace)
LSM late systolic murmur
LSO left salpingo-oophorectomy
left superior oblique
lumbosacral orthosis
LSP left sacrum posterior
liver-specific (membrane) lipoprotein
L–Spar Elspar (asparaginase)
LSR left superior rectus
L/S ratio lecithin/sphingomyelin ratio
LSS liver-spleen scan
LST left sacrum transverse
LSTC laparoscopic tubal coagulation
L.S.T.L. laparoscopic tubal ligation
L's & T's lines and tubes
LSV left subclavian vein
LSVC left superior vena cava
LT laboratory technician
left
left thigh
leukotrienes
levin tube
light
lumbar traction
LTA local tracheal anesthesia
LTB laparoscopic tubal banding
laryngotracheo-bronchitis
LTB_4 leukotriene B_4
LTC left to count
long-term care
LTC_4 leukotriene C_4
LTCF long-term care facility
LTCS low transverse cesarean section
LTD largest tumor dimension
LTG long-term goal
LTGA left transposition of great artery
LTL laparoscopic tubal ligation
LTM long-term memory
LTOT long-term oxygen therapy
LTS laparoscopic tubal sterilization
LTT lactose tolerance test

	lymphocyte transformation test
LTV	Luche tumor virus
LU	living unit
L & U	lower and upper
LUA	left upper arm
LUE	left upper extremity
Lues I	primary syphilis
LUL	left upper lid
	left upper lobe (lung)
LUOB	left upper outer buttock
LUOQ	left upper outer quadrant
LUQ	left upper quadrant
LURD	living unrelated donor
LUSB	left upper sternal border
LV	leave
	left ventricle
	leucovorin
LVA	left ventricular ancurysm
LVAD	left ventricular assist device
L-VAM	leuprolide acetate, vinblastine, doxorubicin, and mitomycin
LVAT	left ventricular activation time
LVD	left ventricular dysfunction
LVDP	left ventricular diastolic pressure
LVDV	left ventricular diastolic volume
LVE	left ventricular enlargement
LVEDP	left ventricular end diastolic pressure
LVEDV	left ventricular end diastolic volume
LVEF	left ventricular ejection fraction
LVEP	left ventricular end pressure
LVESVI	left ventricular end-systolic volume index
LVET	left ventricular ejection time
LVF	left ventricular failure
LVFP	left ventricular filling pressure
LVG	left ventrogluteal
LVH	left ventricular hypertrophy
LVIDd	left ventricle internal dimension diastole
LVIDs	left ventricle internal dimension systole
LVL	left vastus lateralis
LVMM	left ventricular muscle mass
LVN	Licensed Visiting Nurse
	Licensed Vocational Nurse
LVOP	left ventricular outflow tract
LVP	large volume parenteral
	left ventricular pressure
LVPW	left ventricular posterior wall
LVR	leucovorin
LVSEMI	left ventricular subendocardial myocardialischemia
LVSP	left ventricular systolic pressure
LVSWI	left ventricular stroke work index
LVV	left ventricular volume
	live varicella vaccine
LVW	left ventricular wall
LVWI	left ventricular work index
LVWMA	left ventricular wall motion abnormality
LVWMI	left ventricular wall motion index
L & W	living and well
LWCT	Lee-White clotting time
LWBS	left without being seen
LWC	leave without consent
LWP	large whirlpool
lx	larynx
	lower extremity
LXC	laxative of choice
LXT	left exotropia
LYG	lymphmatoid granulomatosis
LYM	lymphocytes

lymphs	lymphocytes
LYS	lysine
lytes	electrolytes (Na, K, Cl, etc.)

M

M	male
	marital
	married
	mass
	medial
	meta
	meter (m)
	million
	minimum
	molar
	Monday
	monocytes
	mother
	mouth
	murmur
	muscle
	myopia
	myopic
	thousand
M	murmur
M_1	first mitral sound
M1	left mastoid
M^2	square meters (body surface)
M2	right mastoid
M-2	vincristine, carmustine, cyclophosphamide, melphalan, and prednisone
MA	machine
	medical assistance
	medical authorization
	menstrual age
	mental age
	Mexican American
	Miller-Abbott (tube)
	milliamps
	monoclonal antibodies
	motorcycle accident
M/A	mood and/or affect
MAA	macroaggregates of albumin
MAB	monoclonal antibody
MABP	mean arterial blood pressure
MAAC	no apparent anesthetic complications
MAC	macrocytic erythrocytes
	macula
	maximal allowable concentration
	methotrexate, dactinomycin, and cyclophosphamide
	mid-arm circumference
	minimum alveolar concentration
	monitored anesthesia care
MACC	methotrexate, doxorubicin, cyclophosphamide, and lomustine
MACOP-B	methotrexate, doxorubicin, cyclophosphamide, vincristine, prednisone, and bleomycin
MACRO	macrocytes
MADRS	Montgomery-Asburg Depression Rating Scale
MAE	moves all extremities
MAEEW	moves all extremities equally well
MAEW	moves all extremities well
MAFAs	movement-associated fetal (heart rate) accelerations
mag cit	magnesium citrate
mag sulf	magnesium sulfate
MAHA	macroangiopathic hemolytic anemia
MAI	maximal aggregation index
	minor acute illness
	Mycobacterium avium-intracellulare
MAL	malignant
	midaxillary line
malig	malignant
MALT	mucosa-associated lymphoid tissue

MAMC mid-arm muscle circumference
Mammo mammography
m-AMSA amsacrine
Mand mandibular
MANOVA multivariate analysis of variance
MAO maximum acid output
MAOI monoamine oxidase inhibitor
MAP mean airway pressure
mean arterial pressure
mitomycin, doxorubicin, and cisplatin
MAPS make a picture story
megaloblastic anemia of pregnancy
MAR medication administration record
MAS meconium aspiration syndrome
mobile arm support
MAST mastectomy
military antishock trousers
MAT manual arts therapy
maternal
maternity
mature
medication administration team
multifocal atrial tachycardia
MAVR mitral and aortic valve replacement
max maxillary
maximal
MB buccal margin
Mallory body
M-BACOD methotrexate, calcium leucovorin, bleomycin, doxorubicin, cyclophosphamide, vincristine, and dexamethasone
MBC maximum bladder capacity
maximum breathing capacity
methotrexate, bleomycin, and cisplatin
minimal bacteriocidal concentration
MB-CK a creatinine kinase isoenzyme
MBC nonbed care
MBEST modulus blipped echo-planar single-pulse technique
MBD minimal brain damage
minimal brain dysfunction
MBE medium below elbow
MBF meat base formula
myocardial blood flow
MBFC medial brachial fascial compartment
MBHH newborn helpful hints
MBI methylene blue installation
MBL menstrual blood loss
MBM mothers breast milk
MBNW multiple-breath nitrogen washout
MBO mesiobuccal occulsion
MC metatarso - cuneiform
mitoxantrone and cytarabine
mixed cellularity
molluscum contagiosum
monocomponent highly purified pork insulin
mouth care
m + c morphine and cocaine
MCA megestrol, cyclophosphamide and doxorubicin
middle cerebral aneurysm
middle cerebral artery
monoclonal antibodies
motorcycle accident
multichannel analyzer
McB pt McBurney's point
MCC midstream clean-catch
MCCU mobile coronary care unit
MCDT mast cell degranulation test
mcg microgram (μg)
MCGN minimal-change glomerular nephritis
MCH mean corpuscular hemoglobin

muscle contraction headache
MCHC mean corpuscular hemoglobin concentration
mCi millicurie
MCL medial collateral ligament
midclavicular line
midcostal line
modified chest lead
most comfortable listening level
MCLNS mucocutaneous lymph node syndrome
MCMI Million Clinical Multiaxial Inventory
mcmol micromoles
MCP metacarpophalangeal joint
metoclopramide
MCS microculture and sensitivity
MCSA minimal crosssectional area
MCT manual cervical traction
mean circulation time
medium chain triglyceride
medullary carcinoma of the thyroid
MCTC metrizamide computer tomography cisternogram
MCTD mixed connective tissue disease
MCU micturating cystourethrogram
MCV mean corpuscular volume
MD maintenance dialysis
major depression
mammary dysplasia
manic depression
medical doctor
mediodorsal
mental deficiency
movement disorder
muscular dystrophy
MDA malondialdehyde
manual dilation of the anus
methylenedioxyamphetamine
motor discriminativeacuity
MDC medial dorsal cutaneous (nerve)
MDD major depressive disorder
manic depressive disorder
MDE major depressive episode
MDF myocardial depressant factor
MDI manic depressive illness
metered dose inhaler
methylenedioxyindenes
multiple daily injection
multiple dosage insulin
MDIA Mental Development Index, Adjusted
MDII multiple daily insulin injection
MDM middiastolic murmur
minor determinant mix (of penicillin)
MDP methylene diphosphonate
MDPI maximum daily permissible intake
MDR minimum daily requirement
MDS maternal deprivation syndrome
myelodysplastic syndromes
MDT multidisciplinary team
MDTM multidisciplinary team meeting
MDTP multidisciplinary treatment plan
MDUO myocardial disease of unknown origin
MDV Marek's disease virus
multiple dose vial
MDY month, date, and year
ME macula edema
manic episode
medical examiner
middle ear
M/E myeloid-erythroid (ratio)
MEA-I multiple endocrine adenomatosis type I
MEB methylene blue
MEC meconium
middle ear canals

MeCCNU semustine

MECG maternal electrocardiogram

MeCP methyl-CCNU, cyclophosphamide, and prednisone

MED medial
median erythrocyte diameter
medical
medication
medicine
medium
minimum effective dose

MEDAC multiple endocrine deficiency-autoimmune-candidiasis

MED-LARS Medical Literature Analysis and Retrieval System

MEE measured energy expenditure
middle ear effusion

MEF maximum expired flow rate
middle ear fluid

MEFR mid expiratory flow rate

MEFV maximum expiratory flow-volume

MEG magnetoenephalogram
magnetoencephalogram

MEL B melarsoprol

men meningeal
meninges
meningitis

MEN (II) memory
multiple endocrine neoplasia (type II)

MEO malignant external otitis

MEOS microsomal ethanol oxidizing system

mEq milliequivalent

mEq/24 H millequivalents per 24 hours

mEq/L milliequivalents per liter

M/E ratio myeloid/erythroid ratio

MEP meperidine

MES mesial

MET medical emergency treatment
metabolic
metastasis

META metamyelocytes

METHb methemoglobin

methyl CCNU semustine

methyl G mitroguazone dihydrochloride

methyl GAG mitroguazone dihydrochloride

MET metamyelocytes

METS metabolic equivalents (multiples of resting oxygen uptake)
metastasis

METT maximum exercise tolerance test

MEV million electron volts

MEX Mexican

MF Malassezia furfur
masculinity/femininity
meat free
methotrexate, fluorouracil and calcium leucovorin
midcavity forceps
mycosis fungoides
myocardial fibrosis

M & F male and female
mother and father

MFAT multifocal atrial tachycardia

MFB metallic foreign body

MFD midforceps delivery
milk-free diet

MFEM maximal forced expiratory maneuver

MFH malignant fibrous histiocytoma

MFR mid-forceps rotation

MFT muscle function test

MFVNS middle fossa vestibular nerve section

MFVPT Motor Free Visual Perception Test

MG Marcus Gunn
milligram (mg)
myasthenia gravis

Mg magnesium

mg% milligrams per 100 milliliters

mg/dl milligrams per 100 milliliters
MGF maternal grandfather
mg/kg milligram per kilogram
mg/kg/d milligram per kilogram per day
mg/kg/hr milligram per kilogram per hour
MGM maternal grandmother
milligram (mg is correct)
MGN membranous glomerulonephritis
MgO magnesium oxide
MGP Marcus-Gunn's pupil
$MgSO_4$ magnesium sulfate (Epsom salt)
MGUS monoclonal gammapathies of undetermined significance
M-GXT multi-stage graded exercise test
MH malignant hyperthermia
marital history
menstrual history
mental health
moist heat
MHA mental health assistant
microangiopathic hemolytic anemia
microhemagglutination
MHB maximum hospital benefit
methemoglobin
MHBSS modified Hank's balanced salt solution
MHC major histocompatibility complex
mental health center
mental health counselor
M/hct microhematocrit
mHg millimeters of mercury
MHI Mental Health Index (information)
MH/MR mental health & mental retardation
MHN massive hepatic necrosis
MHRI Mental Health Research Institute
MHS major histocompatibility system
malignant hyperthermia susceptible
MHW medial heel wedge
mental health worker
MHz megahertz
MI membrane intact
mental illness
mental institution
mitral insufficiency
myocardial infarction
MIA medically indigent adult
missing in action
MIC maternal and infant care
medical intensive care
microscope
microcytic erythrocytes
minimum inhibitory concentration
MICN mobile intensive care nurse
MICR methacholine inhalation challenge response
MICRO microcytes
MICU medical intensive care unit
mobile intensive care unit
MID multi-infarct dementia
Mid I middle insomnia
MIE medical improvement expected
MIF merthiolateiodine-formalin
migration inhibitory factor
MIFR mid-inspiratory flow rate
MIH migraine with interparoxysmal headache
MIL military
mother-in-law
MIN mineral
minimum
minor
minute (min)
MINE mesna uroprotection, ifosfamide, mitoxantrone, and etoposide
MINE medical improvement not expected
MIO minimum identifiable odor

MIP maximum inspiratory pressure
medical improvement possible
metacarpointerphalangeal

MIRD Medical Internal Radiation Dose

MIRP myocardial infarction rehabilitation program

MIS mitral insufficiency

MISC miscarriage
miscellaneous

MISO misonidazole

MISS Modified Injury Severity Score (scale)

MIT meconium in trachea

MITO-C mitomycin

mix mon mixed monitor

MJ marijuana
mega joule

MJT Mead Johnson tube

MK-CSF megakrayocyte colony stimulating-factor

MKAB may keep at bedside

ML middle lobe
midline

mL milliliter

M/L monocyte to lymphocyte (ratio)
mother-in-law

MLA mentolaeva anterior

MLC minimal lethal concentration
mixed lymphocyte culture
multi-level care
multilumen catheter

MLD masking level difference
metachromatic leukodystrophy
minimal lethal dose

MLE midline episiotomy

MLF median longitudinal fasciculus

MLNS mucocutaneous lymph node syndrome

MLR middle latency response
mixed lymphocyte reaction
multiple logistic regression

MLU mean length of utterance

MM malignant melanoma
Marshall-Marchetti
medial malleolus
meningococcic meningitis
mercaptopurine and methotrexate
methadone maintenance
millimeter (mm)
morbidity and mortality
motor meal
mucous membrane
multiple myeloma

mM. millimole

M&M milk and molasses
morbidity and mortality

MMA methylmalonic acid

MMC mitomycin (mitomycin C)

MMECT multiple monitor electroconvulsive therapy

MMEFR maximal midexpiratory flow rate

MMF mean maximum flow

MMFR maximal mid expiratory flow rate

mmHg millimeters of mercury

MMI methimazole

MMK Marshall-Marchetti-Krantz (cystourethroplexy)

MMM myelofibrosis with myeloid metaplasia

MMMT metastatic mixed Müllerian tumor

MMOA maxillary mandibular odentectomy alveolectomy

mmol millimole

MMPI Minnesota Multiphasic Personality Inventory

MMPI-D Minnesota Multiphasic Personality Inventory-Depression Scale

6-MMPR 6 methylmercaptopurine riboside

MMR measles, mumps, and rubella
midline malignant reticulosis

MMS Mini-Mental State (examination)
MMT manual muscle test
Mini Mental Test
MMTP Methadone Maintenance Treatment Program
MMV mandatory minute volume
MMWR Morbidity & Mortality Weekly Report
MN midnight
Mn manganese
M&N morning and night
MNC mononuclear leukocytes
M/NCV motor nerve conduction velocity
MND modified neck dissection
motoneuron disease
MNG multinodular goiter
MNR marrow neutrophil reserve
Mn SSEPS median nerve somato-sensory evoked potentials
MNTB medial nucleus of the trapezoid body
MO medial oblique (x-ray view)
mesio-occlusal
mineral oil
month (mo)
months old
morbidly obese
mother
Mo molybdenum
MOA mechanism of action
MoAb monoclonal antibody
MOB medical office building
MOB-PT mitomycin, vincristine, bleomycin, and cisplatin
MOC mother of child
MOD maturity onset diabetes
medical officer of the day
mesio-occlusodistal
moderate
MODM mature-onset diabetes mellitus
MODY maturity onset diabetes of the youth
MOF methotrexate, vincristine, and fluorouracil
MOFS multiple-organ failure syndrome
MOJAC mood orientation, judgement, affect, and content
MOM milk of magnesia
mucoid otitis media
MON monitor
mono. infectious mononucleosis
monocyte
monospot
MOP medical outpatient
MOPP mechlorethamine, vincristine, procarbazine, and prednisone
MOPV monovalent oral poliovirus vaccine
MOR morphine
MOS mirrow optical system
months
mOsm milliosmole
mOsmol milliosmole
MOT motility examination
MOTT mycobacteria other than tubercle
MOUS multiple occurrences of unexplained symptoms
MOV multiple oral vitamin
MP melphalan and prednisone
menstrual period
mercaptopurine
metacarpal phalangeal joint
moist park
mouthpiece
4MP4 methylpyrazole
6-MP mercaptopurine
MPA main pulmonary artery
medroxyprogesterone acetate
MPAG McGill Pain Assessment Questionnaire
MPAP mean pulmonary artery pressure
MPB male pattern baldness
MPC mucopurulent cervicitis
MPCN microscopically positive, and culturally negative

MPD maximum permissable dose
multiple personality disorder
MPGN membranoproliferative glomerulonephritis
MPH Master of Public Health
methylphenidate
MPJ metacarpophalangeal joint
mpk milligram per kilogram
MPL maximum permissable level
MPM Mortality Prediction Model
MPOA medial preoptic area
MPP massive periretinal proliferation
MPQ McGill Pain Questionnaire
MPPT methylprednisolone pulse therapy
MPS mucopolysaccharidosis
multiphasic screening
MPSS methylprednisolone sodium succinate
MPTR motor, pain, touch, reflex, and deficit
MPV mean platelet volume
MQ memory quotient
MR magnetic resonance
Maddox rod
may repeat
measles-rubella
medial rectus
medical record
mental retardation
milliroentgen
mitral regurgitation
moderate resistance
M&R measure and record
MR × 1 may repeat times one (once)
MRA main renal artery
medical record administrator
mid-right atrium
MRAN medical resident admitting note
MRAP mean right atrial pressure
MRAS main renal artery stenosis
MRD margin reflex distance
Medical Records Department
MRDD Mental Retardation and Development Disabilities
MRDM malnutrition-related diabetes mellitus
MRE manual resistance exercise
MRG murmurs, rubs, and gallops
MRH Maddox rod hyperphoria
MRI magnetic resonance imaging
MRM modified radical mastectomy
mRNA messenger ribonucleic acid
MRS magnetic resonance spectroscopy
methicillin resistant *Staphylococcus aureus*
MRSA methicillin-resistant *Staphylococcus aureus*
MRSE methicillin-resistant *staphylococcus epidermitis*
MS mass spectroscopy
medical student
mental status
milk shake
minimal support
mitral sounds
mitral stenosis
morning stiffness
morphine sulfate
multiple sclerosis
muscle strength
musculoskeletal
M & S microculture and sensitivity
MS III third-year medical student
MSAF meconium stained amniotic fluid
MSAFP maternal serum alpha fetoprotein
MSAP mean systemic arterial pressure
MSBOS maximum surgical blood order schedule

MSCA McCarthy Scales of Children's Abilities
MSCU medical special care unit
MSCWP musculoskeletal chest wall pain
MSD microsurgical discectomy
mid-sleep disturbance
MSE Mental Status Examination
Msec milliseconds
MSEL myasthenic syndrome of Eaton-Lambert
MSER mean systolic ejection rate
Mental Status Examination Record
MSF meconium-stained fluid
megakaryocyte stimulating factor
MSG methysergide
monosodium glutamate
MSH melanocyte-stimulating hormone
MSIR® morphine sulfate immediate release tablets
MSK medullary sponge kidney
MSL midsternal line
MSLT multiple sleep latency test
MSO_4 morphine sulfate (this is a dangerous abbreviation)
MSPN medical student progress notes
MSPU medical short procedure unit
MSR muscle stretch reflexes
MSS Marital Satisfaction Scale
minor surgery suite
muscular subaortic stenosis
MST mean survival time
MSTA® mumps skin test antigen
MSTI multiple soft tissue injuries
MSU maple syrup urine
midstream urine
MSUD maple-syrup urine disease
MSW Master of Social Work
multiple stab wounds
MT empty
malaria therapy
malignant teratoma
medical technologist
metatarsal
muscles and tendons
music therapy
M/T masses of tenderness
myringotomy with tubes
M & T Monilia and Trichomonas
myringotomy and tubes
MTAD tympanic membrane of the left ear
MTAS tympanic membrane of the left ear
MTAU tympanic membranes of both ears
MTB *Mycobacterium tuberculosis*
MTBE methyl tert-butyl ether
MTD Monroe Tidal drainage
MTDI maximum tolerable daily intake
MTET modified treadmill exercise testing
MTG mid-thigh girth
MTI malignant teratoma intermiate
MTM modified Thayer-Martin medium
MTP master treatment plan
medical termination of pregnancy
metatarsal phalangeal
MTR-O no masses, tenderness, or rebound
MTRS Licensed Master Therapeutic Recreation Specialist
MTST maximal treadmill stress test
MTU malignant teratoma undifferentiated
methylthiouracil
MTX methotrexate
MTZ mitoxantrone
MU million units
mU milliunits
MUAC middle upper arm circumference

MUGA	multiple gated acquisition
MUGX	multiple gated acquisition exercise
mus-lig	musculoligamentous
MUU	mouse uterine units
MV	mechanical ventilation
	millivolts
	minute volume
	mitoxantrone and etoposide
	mitral valve
	mixed venous
	multivesicular
MVA	malignant vertricular arrhythmias
	mitral valve area
	motor vehicle accident
M-VAC	methotrexate, vinblastine, doxorubicin, and cisplatin
MVAC	methotrexate, vinblastine, doxorubicin, and cisplatin
MVB	mixed venous blood
MVC	maximal voluntary contraction
MVD	microvascular decompression
	mitral valve disease
	multivessel disease
MVE	mitral valve (leaflet) excursion
MVI	multiple vitamin injection
MVI®	trade name for parenteral multivitamins
MVI 12®	trade name for parenteral multivitamins
MVO_2	myocardial oxygen consumption
MVP	mean venous pressure
	mitral valve prolapse
MVPP	mechlorethamine, vinblastine, procarbazine, and prednisone
MVR	massive vitreous retraction
	mitral valve regurgitation
	mitral valve replacement
MVS	mitral valve stenosis
	motor, vascular, and sensory
MVV	maximum voluntary ventilation
	mixed vespid venom
MWD	microwave diathermy
MWI	Medical Walk-In (Clinic)
MWS	Mickety-Wilson syndrome
MWT	malpositioned wisdom teeth
Mx	myringotomy
My	myopia
myelo	myelocytes
	myelogram
MYD	mydriatic
MyG	myasthenia gravis
MZ	monozygotic
MZL	marginal zone lymphocyte

N

N	negative
	Negro
	nerve
	never
	no
	nodes
	normal
	not
	noun
	NPH insulin
	size of sample
N_2	nitrogen
5′-N	5′-Nucleotidase
Na	sodium
NA	Native American
	Narcotics Anonymous
	Negro adult
	nicotinic acid
	not admitted
	not applicable
	not available
	nurse aide
	Nurse Anesthetist
	nursing assistant
N & A	normal and active
NAA	neutron activation analysis
	no apparent abnormalities

NABS normoactive bowel sounds
NaClO sodium hypochlorite
NaCl sodium chloride (salt)
NAD no active disease
no acute distress
no apparent distress
no appreciable disease
normal axis deviation
nothing abnormal detected
NADPH nicotinamide adenine dinucleotide phosphate
NADSIC no apparent disease seen in chest
NaF sodium fluoride
NAF nafcillin
Negro adult female
NAG narrow angle glaucoma
$NaHCO_3$ sodium bicarbonate
NAI no acute inflammation
non-accidental injury
NaI sodium iodide
NANB non-A, non-B (hepatitis)
NAP narrative, assessment, and plan
NAPA N-acetyl procainamide
NAPD no active pulmonary disease
Na Pent Pentothal Sodium®
NAR not at risk
NARC narcotic(s)
NAS nasal
neonatal abstinence syndrome
no added salt
NAT no action taken
NB nail bed
needle biopsy
newborn
nitrogen balance
note well
NBD neurologic bladder dysfunction
no brain damage
NBF not breast fed
NBI no bone injury
NBICU newborn intensive care unit
NBM no bowel movement
normal bone marrow
normal bowel movement
nothing by mouth
NBN newborn nursery
NBP needle biopsy of prostate
NBQC narrow base quad cane
NBS newborn screen (serum thyroxine and phenylketonuria)
no bacteria seen
normal bowel sound
NBT nitroblue tetrazolium reduction (tests)
NBTE nonbacterial thrombotic endocarditis
NBTNF newborn, term, normal female
NBTNM newborn, term, normal, male
NC nasal cannula
Negro child
neurologic check
no change
no charge
no complaints
noncontributory
nose clips
not completed
not cultured
NCA neurocirculatory asthenia
no congenital abnormalities
NCAS neocarzinostatin
NC/AT normal cephalic atraumatic
NCB no code blue
NCC no concentrated carbohydrates
NCD normal childhood diseases
not considered disabling
NCF neutrophilic chemotactic factor
NCI National Cancer Institute
NCJ needle catheter jejunostomy
NCL neuronal ceroid lipofuscinosis
nuclear cardiology laboratory
NCM nailfold capillary microscope

NCNC	normochromic, normocytic
NCO	no complaints offered
	non-commissioned officer
NCP	nursing care plan
NCPAP	nasal continuous positive airway pressure
NCPR	no cardiopulmonary resuscitation
NCRC	non-child resistant container
NCS	nerve conduction studies
	no concentrated sweets
	zinostatis (neocarzinostatin)
NCT	neutron capture therapy
	noncontact tonometry
NCV	nerve conduction velocity
ND	nasal deformity
	natural death
	neurological development
	no disease
	nondisabling
	none detectable
	normal delivery
	normal development
	nose drops
	not diagnosed
	not done
	nothing done
N&D	nodular and diffuse
Nd	neodymium
NDA	New Drug Application
	no data available
	no detectable activity
NDD	no dialysis days
NDI	neurogenic diabetes insipidus
Nd/NT	nondistended, nontender
NDP	net dietary protein
NDR	neurotic depressive reaction
	normal detrusor reflex
NDT	neurodevelopmental treatment
	noise detection threshold
NDV	Newcastle disease virus
NE	never exposed
	no effect
	no enlargement
	norepinephrine
	not elevated
	not examined
NEC	necrotizing entercolitis
	not elsewhere classified
NED	no evidence of disease
NEEP	negative end-expiratory pressure
NEF	negative expiratory force
NEFA	non-esterified fatty acids
NEG	negative
	neglect
NEPHRO	nephrogram
NEM	no evidence of malignancy
NEMD	nonspecific esophageal motility disorder
NEOH	neonatal high risk
NEOM	neonatal medium risk
NEP	no evidence of pathology
NER	no evidence of recurrence
NERD	no evidence of recurrent disease
NES	not elsewhere specified
NET	naso-endotracheal tube
NETT	nasal endotracheal tube
NEX	nose to ear to xiphoid
NF	Negro female
	neurofibromatosis
	none found
	not found
	nursed fair
NFD	no family doctor
NFL	nerve fiber layer
NFP	no family physician
NFTD	normal full term delivery
NFTSD	normal full-term spontaneous delivery
NFTT	nonorganic failure to thrive
NFW	nursed fairly well
NG	nanogram
	nasogastric
	nitroglycerin
	no growth
NGB	neurogenic bladder
NGF	nerve growth factor
n giv	not given
NGR	nasogastric replacement

NGRI	not guilty by reason of insanity
NGT	nasogastric tube
	normal glucose tolerance
NGU	nongonococcal urethritis
NH	nursing home
NHC	neighborhood health center
	neonatal hypocalcemia
	nursing home care
NH_3	ammonia
NH_4Cl	ammonium chloride
NHCU	nursing home care unit
NHD	normal hair distribution
NHL	nodular histiocytic lymphoma
	non-Hodgkin's lymphomas
nHL	normalized hearing level
NHP	nursing home placement
NI	neurological improvement
	no information
	not identified
	not isolated
NIA	no information available
NIAL	not in active labor
NICC	neonatal intensive care center
NICU	neonatal intensive care unit
	neurosurgical intensive care unit
NIDD	non-insulin-dependent diabetes
NIDDM	non-insulin-dependent diabetes mellitus
NIF	negative inspiratory force
	not in file
NIG	NSAIA (non-steroidal anti-inflamatory agent) induced gastropathy
NIH	National Institutes of Health
NIHL	noise-induced hearing loss
NIL	not in labor
NIMHDIS	National Institute for Mental Health Diagnostic Interview Schedule
NINU	neuro intermediate nursing unit
NINVS	non-invasive neurovascular studies
NIP	no infection present
	no inflammation present
Nitro	nitroglycerin (this is a dangerous abbreviation)
	sodium nitroprusside
NJ	nasojejunal
NK	natural killer (cells)
	not known
NKA	no known allergies
NKC	nonketotic coma
NKDA	no known drug allergies
NKFA	no known food allergies
NKHA	nonketotic hyperosmolar acidosis
NKHS	nonketotic hyperosmolar syndrome
NKMA	no known medication allergies
NL	nasolacrimal
	normal
NLB	needle liver biopsy
NLC & C	normal libido, coitus, and climax
NLD	nasolacrimal duct
	necrobiosis lipoidica diabeticorum
NLE	nursing late entry
NLF	nasolabial fold
NLP	no light perception
	nodular liquifying panniculitis
NLS	neonatal lupus syndrome
NLT	not later than
	not less than
NM	neuromuscular
	Negro male
	nodular melanoma
	nonmalignant
	not measurable
	not measured
	not mentioned
	nuclear medicine
N & M	nerves and muscles
	night and morning
NMD	normal muscle development

NMI	no mental illness
	no middle initial
	normal male infant
NMN	no middle name
nmol	nanomole
NMP	normal menstrual period
NMR	nuclear magnetic resonance (same as magnetic resonance imaging)
NMS	neuroleptic malignant syndrome
NMSE	normalized mean square root
NMSIDS	near-miss sudden infant death syndrome
NMT	nebulized mist treatment
	no more than
NMTB	neuromuscular transmission blockade
NN	neonatal
	normal nursery
	nurses' notes
N/N	negative/negative
NND	neonatal death
NNE	neonatal necrotizing enterocolitis
NNM	Nicolle-Novy-MacNeal (media)
NNL	no new laboratory (test orders)
NNO	no new orders
NNP	Neonatal Nurse Practitioner
NNS	neonatal screen (hematocrit, total bilirubin, and total protein)
NNU	net nitrogen utilization
NO	nasal oxygen
	nitrous oxide
	none obtained
	nonobese
	number (no.)
	nursing office
N_2O	nitrous oxide
$N_2O:O_2$	nitrous oxide to oxygen ratio
noc.	night
noct	nocturnal
NOD	nonobese diabetic
	notify of death
NOK	next of kin
NOM	nonsuppurative otitis media
NOMI	nonocclusive mesenteric infarction
non pal	not palpable
NOOB	not out of bed
NOR	normal
	nortriptyline
NOR-EPI	norepinephrine
norm	normal
NOS	not on staff
	not otherwise specified
NOSIE	Nurse's Observation Scale for Inpatient Evaluation
NOT	nocturnal oxygen therapy
NP	nasal prongs
	nasopharyngeal
	near point
	neurophysin
	neuropsychiatric
	newly presented
	nonpalpable
	no pain
	not performed
	not pregnant
	not present
	nursed poorly
	nuclear pharmacist
	nuclear pharmacy
	nurse practitioner
NPA	nasal pharyngeal airway
	near point of accommodation
NPAT	nonparoxysmal atrial tachycardia
NPC	near point convergences
	nodal premature contractions
	nonpatient contact
	nonpro ductive cough
	nonprotein calorie
NPDL	nodular poorly differentiated lymphocytic
NPDR	nonproliferative diabetic retinopathy

NPE	neuropsychologic examination
	no palpable enlargement
	normal pelvic examination
NPF	nasopharyngeal fiberscope
	no predisposing factor
NPH	a type of insulin (Isophane)
	no previous history
	normal pressure hydrocephalus
NPG	nonpregnant
NPhx	nasopharynx
NPI	no present illness
NPJT	nonparoxysmal junctional tachycardia
NPN	nonprotein nitrogen
NPO	nothing by mouth
NPP	normal postpartum
NPPNG	nonpenicillinase-producing *Neisseria gonorrhoeae*
NPR	normal pulse rate
	nothing per rectum
NPSA	nonphysician surgical assistant
NPT	nocturnal penile tumescence
	normal pressure and temperature
NPU	net protein utilization
NQMI	non-Q wave myocardial infarction
NR	do not repeat
	no refills
	no report
	no response
	no return
	nonreactive
	nonrebreathing
	normal range
	normal reaction
	not reached
NRAF	non-rheumatic atrial fibrillation
NRBC	normal red blood cell
	nucleated red blood cell
NRBS	non-rebreathing system
NRC	National Research Council
	normal retinal correspondence
	Nuclear Regulatory Commission
NREM	nonrapid eye movement
NREMS	nonrapid eye movement sleep
NRF	normal renal function
NRI	nerve root involvement
	nerve root irritation
NRM	normal range of motion
	normal retinal movement
NRN	no return necessary
NROM	normal range of motion
NRT	neuromuscular reeducation techniques
NS	nephrotic syndrome
	neurological signs
	neurosurgery
	nipple stimulation
	nonsmoker
	normal saline solution (0.9% sodium chloride solution)
	no sample
	not seen
	not significant
	nuclear sclerosis
	nylon suture
N $\bar{s}$ E	nausea without emesis
NSA	no salt added
	no significant abnormality
	normal serum albumin
NSABP	National Surgical Adjuvant Breast Project
NSAD	no signs of acute disease
NSAIA	non-steroidal antiinflammatory agent
NSAID	non-steroidal antiinflammatory drug
NSC	no significant change
	not service-connected
NSCD	nonservice-connected disability
NSCLC	non-small-cell lung cancer
NSD	no significant disease (difference, defect, deviation)

	nominal standard dose
	normal spontaneous delivery
NSDA	non-steroid dependent asthmatic
NSE	neuron-specific enolase
	normal saline enema (0.9% sodium chloride)
NSFTD	normal spontaneous full-term delivery
NSG	nursing
NSI	negative self-image
	no signs of infection
	no signs of inflammation
NSILA	nonsuppressible insulin-like activity
NSN	nephrotoxic serum nephritis
NSO	Neosporin® ointment
NSP	neck and shoulder pain
NSPVT	nonsustained polymorphic ventricular tachycardia
NSR	nasoseptal repair
	nonspecific reaction
	normal sinus rhythm
	not seen regularly
NSS	normal size and shape
	not statistically significant
	nutritional support service
	sodium chloride 0.9% (normal saline solution)
1/2 NSS	sodium chloride 0.45% (1/2 normal saline solution)
NSSL	normal size, shape, and location
NSSP	normal size, shape, and position
NSSTT	nonspecific ST and T (wave)
NSST-TWCS	nonspecific ST-T wave changes
NST	non-stress test
	not sooner than
	nutritional support team
NSTT	nonseminomatous testicular tumors
NSU	neurosurgical unit
	nonspecific urethritis
NSV	nonspecific vaginitis
NSVD	normal spontaneous vaginal delivery
NSX	neurosurgical examination
NSY	nursery
NT	nasotracheal
	normal temperature
	nortriptyline
	not tender
	not tested
	nourishment taken
N&T	nose and throat
NTBR	not to be resuscitated
NTC	neurotrauma center
NTD	neural tube defects
NTE	not to exceed
NTF	normal throat flora
NTG	nitroglycerin
	nontoxic goiter
	nontreatment group
NTGO	nitroglycerin ointment
NTM	nocturnal tumescence monitor
NTMB	nontuberculous myobacteria
NTMI	non-transmural myocardial infarction
NTND	not tender, not distended
NTP	Nitropaste® (nitroglycerin ointment)
	normal temperature and pressure
	sodium nitroprusside
NTS	nasotracheal suction
	nucleus tractus solitarii
NTT	nasotracheal tube
NU	name unknown
NUD	nonulcer dyspepsia
NUG	necrotizing ulcerative gingivitis
nullip	nullipara
NV	nausea and vomiting
	near vision
	neurovascular
	next visit
	nonvaccinated
	nonvenereal
	nonveteran
	normal value
	not verified
N&V	nausea and vomiting

NVA	near visual acuity
NVAF	nonvalvular atrial fibrillation
NVD	nausea, vomiting, and diarrhea
	neck vein distention
	neovascularization of the disc
	neurovesicle dysfunction
	no venereal disease
	nonvalvular disease
NVE	neovascularization elsewhere
NVG	neovascular glaucoma
	neoviridogrisein
NVL	neurovascular laboratory
NVS	neurological vital signs
NVSS	normal variant short stature
NW	naked weight
	nasal wash
	not weighed
NWB	non-weight bearing
NWC	number of words chosen
NWD	neuroleptic withdrawal
Nx	nephrectomy
NYD	not yet diagnosed
NYHA	New York Heart Association (classification of heart disease)
nyst	nystagmus
NZ	enzyme

O

O	eye
	objective findings
	obvious
	occlusal
	often
	open
	oral
	ortho
	other
	oxygen
	pint
	zero
ō	negative
	none
	pint
	without
$_1O_2$	singlet oxygen
O_2	both eyes
	oxygen
O_{2v}	superoxide
OA	occiput anterior
	oral airway
	oral alimentation
	osteoarthritis
	Overeaters Anonymous
O & A	observation & assessment
	odontectomy and alveoloplasty
OAC	oral anticoagulant(s)
	overaction
OAD	obstructive airway disease
	occlusive arterial disease
OAE	otoacoustic emissions
OAF	osteoclast activating factor
OAG	open angle glaucoma
OASDHI	Old Age, Survivors, Disability, and Health Insurance
OASO	overactive superior oblique
OASR	overactive superior rectus
OAW	oral airway
OB	obese
	obstetrics
	occult blood
OBE-CALP	placebo capsule or tablet
OBG	obstetrics and gynecology
Ob-Gyn	obstetrics and gynecology
Obj	objective
obl	oblique
OBRR	obstetric recovery room
OBS	obstetrical service
	organic brain syndrome
OBT	obtained
OC	obstetrical conjugate
	office call
	on call
	only child
	oral care
	oral contraceptive
O & C	onset and course
OCA	oculocutaneous albinism

open care area
oral contraceptive agent

OCAD occlusive carotid artery disease

OCC occlusal

OCCC open chest cardiac compression

occl occlusion

OCCM open chest cardiac massage

OCC PR open-chest cardiopulmonary resuscitation

OCC Th occupational therapy

Occup Rx occupational therapy

OCD obsessive-compulsive disorder
osteochondritis dissecans

OCG oral cholecystogram

OCL® oral colonic lavage

OCP oral contraceptive pills
ova, cysts, parasites

11-OCS 11-oxycorticosteroid

OCT ornithine carbamyl transferase
oxytocin challenge test

OCU observation care unit

OD doctor of optometry
Officer-of-the-Day
once daily (this is a dangerous abbreviation as it is read as right eye)
on duty
optic disc
outdoor
overdose
right eye

Δ OD 450 deviation of optical density at 450

ODA occipitodextra anterior
osmotic driving agent

ODAC on demand analgesia computer

ODAT one day at a time

ODC ornithine decarboxylase
outpatient diagnostic center

ODCH ordinary diseases of childhood

ODM ophthalmodynamometry

ODN optokinetic nystagmus

ODP occipitodextra transerve
offspring of diabetic parents

OE on examination
orthopedic examination
otitis externa

O&E observation and examination

OEC outer ear canal

OER oxygen enhancement ratios

OET oral esophageal tube

OETT oral endotracheal tube

OF occipital-frontal
optic fundi

OFC occipital-frontal circumference
orbitofacial cleft

OG Obstetrics-Gynecology
orogastric (feeding)

OGTT oral glucose tolerance test

OH occupational history
on hand
open heart
oral hygiene
orthostatic hypotension
outside hospital

17 OH 17-hydroxycorticosteroids

OHA oral hypoglycemic agents

OH Cbl hydroxycobalamine

17-OHCS 17-hydroxycorticosteroids

OHD hydroxy vitamin D
organic heart disease

OHF omsk hemorrhagic fever
overhead frame

OHG oral hypoglycemic

OHI oral hygiene instructions

OHIAA hydroxyindolacetic acid

OHL oral hairy leukoplakia

OHP oxygen under hyperbaric pressure

OHRR open heart recovery room

OHS occupational health service
ocular hypoperfusion syndrome
open heart surgery

OI opportunistic infection
osteogenesis imperfecta

	otitis interna
OIF	oil-immersion field
OIH	orthoiodohippurate
OIHA	orthoiodohippuric acid
OJ	orange juice (this is a dangerous abbreviation)
	orthoplast jacket
OK	all right
	approved
	correct
OKAN	optokinetic after nystagmus
OKN	optokinetic nystagmus
OL	left eye
OLA	occiput left anterior
OLP	occipitolaevoanterior
OLR	otology, laryngology, and rhinology
OLT	occipitolaevoposterior
	orthotopic liver transplantation
OLTx	orthotopic liver transplantation
OM	every morning (this is a dangerous abbreviation)
	obtuse marginal
	osteomalacia
	osteomyelitis
	otitis media
OMAS	otitis media, acute, suppurating
OMCA	otitis media, catarrhalis, acute
OMCC	otitis media, catarrhalis, chronic
OME	office of Medical Examiner
	otitis media with effusion
7-OMEN	menogaril
OMH	organic marine hydrocolloid
OMI	old myocardial infarct
OMPA	otitis media, purulent, acute
OMPC	otitis media, purulent, chronic
OMR	operative mortality rate
OMSA	otitis media secretory (or suppurative) acute
OMSC	otitis media secretory (or suppurative) chronic
OMVC	open mitral valve commissurotomy
OMVI	operating motor vehicle intoxicated
ON	every night (this is a dangerous abbreviation)
	optic neurophathy
	oronasal
	Ortho-Novum®
	otic nerve
	overnight
ONC	over-the-needle catheter
ONH	optic nerve head
	optic nerve hypoplasia
ONTR	orders not to resuscitate
OO	oral order
o/o	on account of
OOB	out of bed
OOBBRP	out of bed with bathroom privileges
OOC	onset of contractions
	out of cast
	out of control
OOH&NS	ophthalmology, otorhinolaryngology, and head and neck surgery
OOL	onset of labor
OOLR	ophthalmology, otology, laryngology, and rhinology
OOP	out of pelvis
	out of plaster
	out on pass
OOR	out of room
OOS	out of stock
OOT	out of town
OOW	out of wedlock
OP	oblique presentation
	occiput posterior
	open
	operation
	oropharynx
	oscillatory potentials
	osteoporosis
	outpatient
O&P	ova and parasites

OPA	outpatient anesthesia
	oral pharyngeal airway
OPB	outpatient basis
OPC	outpatient clinic
OPCA	olivopontocerebellar atrophy
op cit	in the work cited
OPD	outpatient department
O'p'-DDD	mitotane
OPE	outpatient evaluation
OPG	ocular plethysmography
OPM	occult primary malignancy
OPP	opposite
OPPG	oculopneumoplethysmography
OPS	operations
	outpatient surgery
OPT	optimum
	outpatient treatment
OPT c O_2	Ohio pediatric tent with oxygen
OPT c CA	Ohio pediatric tent with compressed air
OPV	oral polio vaccine
OR	oil retention
	open reduction
	operating room
ORCH	orchiectomy
ORIF	open reduction internal fixation
ORL	otorhinolaryngology
ORN	operating room nurse
OROS	ostomotic release oral system
ORP	occiput right posterior
ORS	oral rehydration salts
ORT	operating room technician
	Registered Occupational Therapist
OR XI	oriented to time
OR X2	oriented to time and place
OR X3	oriented to time, place, and person
OS	left eye
	mouth (this is a dangerous abbreviation as it is read as left eye)
	occipitosacral
	opening snap
	oral surgery
	osmium
OSA	obstructive sleep apnea
OSAS	obstructive sleep apnea syndrome
OSD	overside drainage
OSFT	outstretched fingertips
OSHA	Occupational Safety & Health Administration
OSM S	osmolarity serum
OSM U	osmolarity urine
OSN	off service note
OSS	osseous
	over-shoulder strap
OT	occiput transverse
	occupational therapy
	old tuberculin
OTA	open to air
OTC	ornithonetranscarbamoylase
	over the counter (sold without prescription)
OTD	out the door
OTH	other
OTO	otology
OTR	Occupational Therapist, Registered
OT/RT	occupational therapy/recreational therapy
OTS	orotracheal suction
OTT	orotracheal tube
OU	both eyes
OURQ	outer upper right quadrant
OV	office visit
	ovary
	ovum
OVAL	ovalocytes
OW	once weekly (this is a dangerous abbreviation)
	outer wall
	out of wedlock
OWNK	out of wedlock not keeping
Oxi	oximeter (oximetry)
OXZ	oxazepam
oz	ounce

P

P	para
	peripheral
	phosphorus
	pint
	plan
	protein
	pulse
	pupil
p̄	after
/P	partial lower denture
P/	partial upper denture
P_2	pulmonic second heart sound
^{32}P	radioactive phosphorus
PA	paranoid
	pernicious anemia
	phenol alcohol
	physician assistant
	pineapple
	posterior-anterior (x-ray)
	presents again
	professional association
	psychiatric aide
	pulmonary artery
P&A	percussion and auscultation
	position and alignment
$P_2>A_2$	pulmonic second heart sound greater than aortic secondheart sound
PAB	premature atrial beat
PAC	premature atrial contraction
PACH	pipers to after coming head
$PaCO_2$	arterial carbon dioxide tension
PAC-V	cisplatin, doxorubicin, and cyclophosphamide
PACU	post anesthesia care unit
PAD	primary affective disorder
PADP	pulmonary artery diastolic pressure
PAE	postanoxic encephalopathy
	postantibiotic effect
	progressive assistive exercise
PAEDP	pulmonary artery and end-diastole pressure
PAF	paroxysmal atrial fibrillation
	platelet activating factor
PA&F	percussion, auscultation, and fremitus
PAGA	premature appropriate for gestational age
PAGE	polyacrylamide gel electrophoresis
PAH	para-aminohippurate
	pulmonary arterial hypertension
PAI	plasminogen activator inhibitor
	platelet accumulation index
PAIVS	pulmonary atresia with intact ventricle septum
PAL	posterior axillary line
Pa Line	pulmonary artery line
PALN	para-aortic lymph node
PALS	pediatric advanced life support
PAM	penicillin aluminum monostearate
2-PAM	pralidoxime
PAMP	pulmonary arterial (artery) mean pressure
PAN	periodic alternating nystagmus
	polyarteritis nodosa
PANESS	physical and neurological examination for soft signs
PAO_2	arterial oxygen tension
PAO	peak acid output
PAOP	pulmonary artery occlusion pressure
PAP	passive aggressive personality
	peroxidase-anti-peroxidase
	prostatic acid phosphatase
	pulmonary artery pressure
Pap smear	Papanicolaou smear
PA/PS	pulmonary atresia/pulmonary stenosis

PAR	parafin
	parallel
	platelet aggregate ratio
	postanesthetic recovery
	pulmonary arteriolar resistance
PARA	number of pregnancies
para	paraplegic
PAROM	passive assistance range of motion
PARR	postanesthesia recovery room
PARU	postanesthetic recovery unit
PAS	periodic acid-Schiff (reagent)
	peripheral anterior synechia
	pneumatic antiembolic stocking
	postanesthesia score
	premature auricular systole
	Professional Activities Study
	pulmonary artery stenosis
PAS or PASA	para-aminosalicyclic acid
Pas Ex	passive exercise
PASG	pneumatic antishock garment
PASP	pulmonary artery systolic pressure
PAT	paroxysmal atrial tachycardia
	patella
	patient
	percent acceleration time
	preadmission testing
	pregnancy at term
Path.	pathology
PAV	Pavulon®
PAWP	pulmonary artery wedge pressure
PB	parafin bath
	power building
	powder board
	premature beat
	protein-bound
Pb	lead
	phenobarbital
P&B	pain and burning
	phenobarbital & belladonna
PBA	percutaneous bladder aspiration
PBC	point of basal convergence
	primary biliary cirrhosis
PBD	percutaneous biliary drainage
PBE	partial breech extraction
PBF	placental blood flow
	pulmonary blood flow
PBG	porphobilinogen
PBI	protein-bound iodine
PBK	pseudophakic bullous keratopathy
PBL	peripheral blood lymphocyte
PBMC	peripheral blood mononuclear cell
PBMNC	peripheral blood mononuclear cell
PBN	polymyxin B sulfate, bacitracin, and neomycin
PBO	placebo
PBPI	penile-brachial pulse index
PBS	phosphate-buffered saline
PBT_4	protein-bound thyroxine
PBV	percutaneous balloon valvuloplasty
PBZ	phenoxybenzamine
	phenylbutazone
	pyribenzamine
ΦBZ	phenylbutazone
PC	after meals
	packed cells
	platelet concentrate
	poor condition
	popliteal cyst
	posterior chamber
	present complaint
	productive cough
	professional corporation
PCA	passive cutaneous anaphylaxis

	patient care assistant (aide)
	patient controlled analgesia
	postconceptional age
	posterior cerebral artery
	posterior communicating artery
	procainamide
	procoagulation activity
PCB	pancuronium bromide
	para cervical block
	prepared childbirth
PCBs	polychlorinated biphensyls
PCC	pheochromocytoma
	poison control center
PCCC	pediatric critical care center
PCCU	post coronary care unit
PCD	postmortem cesarean delivery
PCE	physical capacities evaluation
PCE®	erythromycin particles in tablets
PCFT	platelet complement fixation test
PCG	phonocardiogram
PCGG	percutaneous coagulation of gasserian ganglion
PCH	paroxysmal cold hemoglobinuria
PC&HS	after meals and at bedtime
PCI	prophylactic cranial irradiation
PCIOL	posterior chamber intraocular lens
PCKD	polycystic kidney disease
PCL	posterior chamber lens
	posterior cruciate ligament
PCM	protein-calorie malnutrition
PCMX	chloroxylenol
PCN	penicillin
	percutaneous nephrostomy
PCO	polycystic ovary
PCO_2	carbon dioxide pressure (or tension)
PCOD	polycystic ovarian disease
PCP	patient care plan
	phencyclidine
	pneumonocystis carinii pneumonia
	primary care person
	primary care physician
	pulmonary capillary pressure
PCR	polymerase chain reaction
	protein catabolic rate
PCS	patient care system
	portable cervical spine
	portacaval shunt
	postconcussion syndrome
P c/s	primary cesarean section
PCT	porphyria cutanea tarda
	post coital test
	progestin challenge test
PCU	palliative care unit
	primary care unit
	progressive care unit
	protective care unit
PCV	packed cell volume
PCWP	pulmonary capillary wedge pressure
PCX	paracervical
PCXR	portable chest radiograph
PCZ	procarbazine
	prochlorperazine
PD	interpupillary distance
	Parkinson's disease
	percutaneous drain
	peritoneal dialysis
	personality disorder
	poorly differentiated
	postural drainage
	prism diopter
P/D	packs per day (cigarettes)
PDA	parenteral drug abuser
	patent ductus arteriosus
PDD	cisplatin
PDE	paroxysmal dyspnea on exertion
	pulsed Doppler echocardiography
PDFC	premature dead female child

PDGF	platelet derived growth factor
PDGXT	predischarge graded exercise test
PDL	poorly differentiated lymphocytic
	progressively diffused leukoencephalopathy
PDL-D	poorly differentiated lymphocytic-diffuse
PDL-N	poorly differentiated lymphocytic-nodular
PDMC	premature dead male child
PDN	prednisone
	private duty nurse
PD & P	postural drainage and percussion
PDR	Physician's Desk Reference
	postdelivery room
	proliferative diabetic retinopathy
PDRcVH	proliferative diabetic retinopathy with vitreous hemorrhage
PDS	pain dysfunction syndrome
PDT	photodynamic therapy
PDU	pulsed Doppler ultrasonography
PE	cisplatin and etoposide
	physical examination
	physical exercise
	plasma exchange
	plural effusion
	polyethylene
	pressure equalization
	pulmonary edema
	pulmonary embolism
P_1E_1®	epinephrine 1%, pilocarpine 1% ophthalmic solution
PEA	pelvic examination under anesthesia
PEARLA	pupils equal and react to light and accommodation
PEB	cisplatin, etoposide, and bleomycin
PECHO	prostatic echogram
$PECO_2$	mixed expired carbon dioxide tension
Peds.	pediatrics
PEEP	positive end-expiratory pressure
PEFR	peak expiratory flow rate
PEG	percutaneous endoscopic gastrostomy
	pneumoencephalogram
	polyethylene glycol
PEG-ELS	polyethylene glycol and iso-osmolar electrolyte solution
PEGG	Parent Education and Guidance Group
PEJ	percutaneous endoscopic jejunostomy
PEM	protein-energy malnutrition
PEMA	phenylethylmalonamide
PEMS	physical, emotional, mental, and safety
PEN	parenteral and enteral nutrition
PENS	percutaneous epidural nerve stimulator
PEP	pre-ejection period
	protein electrophoresis
PER	by pediatric emergency room
	protein efficiency ratio
PERC	perceptual
	percutaneous
perf.	perfect
	perforation
Peri Care	perineum care
PERL	pupils equal, reactive to light
per os	by mouth (this is a dangerous abbreviation as it is read as left eye)
PERR	pattern evoked retinal response
PERRLA	pupils, equal, round, reactive to light and accommodation
PERRRLA	pupils equal, round, regular, react to light and accommodation

PES	pre-excitation syndrome
	pseudoexpoliation syndrome
peSPL	peak equivalent sound pressure level
PET	poor exercise tolerance
	positron-emission tomography
	pre-eclamptic toxemia
	pressure equalizing tubes
PETN	pentaerythritol tetranitrate
PEx	physical examination
PF	peripheral fields
	plantar flexion
	power factor
	preservative free
	prostatic fluid
PF3	platelet factor 3
PFA	foscarnet (phosphonoformatic acid)
PFC	persistent fetal circulation
PFFFP	Pall filtered fresh frozen plasma
PFJS	patellofemoral joint syndrome
PFM	porcelain fused to metal
PFO	patent foramen ovule
PFPC	Pall filtered packed cells
PFR	parotid flow rate
	peak flow rate
PFRC	plasma-free red cells
PFT	pulmonary function test
PFU	plaque-forming unit
PFW	pHisoHex® face wash
PFWB	Pall filtered whole blood
PG	paged in hospital
	paregoric
	phosphatidyl glycerol
	polygalacturonate
	pregnant
PGA	prostaglandin A
PGE	posterior gastroenterostomy
PGE2	prostaglandin E2
PGF	paternal grandfather
PGF2 α	prostaglandin F2 α
PGH	pituitary growth hormones
PGI	potassium, glucose, and insulin
PGI_2	epoprostenol
PGL	persistent generalized lymphadenopathy
PGM	paternal grandmother
PGP	paternal grandparent
PgR	progesterone receptor
PGU	postgonococcal urethritis
PGY-1	post-graduate year one
*p*H	hydrogen ion concentration
PH	past history
	personal history
	pinhole
	poor health
	pubic hair
	public health
Ph^1	Philadelphia chromosome
PHA	arterial pH
	passive hemagglutinating
	peripheral hyperalimentation
	phytohemagglutinin
	phytohemagglutinin antigen
PHAR	pharmacist
	pharmacy
	pharynx
Pharm	Pharmacy
PharmD	Doctor of Pharmacy
PHC	primary hepatocellular carcinoma
PhD	Doctor of Philosophy
PHH	posthemorrhagic hydrocephalus
PHI	prehospital index
PHIS	posthead injury syndrome
PHL	Philadelphia (chromosome)
PHN	post herpetic neuralgia
	public health nurse
PHPT	primary hyperparathyroidism
PHPV	persistent hyperplastic primary vitreous
PHS	partial hospitalization program
	US Public Health Service
PHT	phenytoin
	portal hypertension
	primary hyperthyroidism
	pulmonary hypertension

PHx past history

Phx pharynx

PI package insert
pancreatic insufficiency
peripheral iridectomy
poison ivy
postinjury
premature infant
present illness
pulmonary infarction

PIAT Peabody Individual Achievement Test

PIC peripherally inserted catheter

PICA Porch Index of Communicative Ability
posterior inferior cerebellar artery
posterior inferior communicating artery

PICC peripherally inserted central catheter

PICU pediatric intensive care unit

PID pelvic inflammatory disease
prolapsed intervertebral disc

PIE pulmonary infiltration with eosinophilia
pulmonary interstitial emphysema

PIF peak inspiratory flow

PIFG poor intrauterine fetal growth

PIG pertussis immune globulin

PIGI pregnancy-induced glucose intolerance

PIH pregnancy induced hypertension

PIMS programmable implantable medication system

PIO pemoline

PIOK poikilocytosis

PI-PB performance intensity-phonemically balanced

PIP peak inspiratory pressure
postinfusion phlebitis
proximal interphalangeal (joint)

PISA phase invariant signature algorithm

Pit patellar inhibition test
Pitocin®
Pitressin® (this is a dangerous abbreviation)
pituitary

PITP pseudo-idiopathic thrombocytopenic purpura

PITR plasma iron turnover rate

PIV peripheral intravenous

PIVD protruded intervertebral disc

PIWT partially impacted wisdom teeth

PJB premature junctional beat

PJC premature junctional contractions

PJS peritoneojugular shunt
Peutz-Jeghers syndrome

PK penetrating keratoplasty

PKB prone knee bend

PKD polycystic kidney disease

PKP penetrating keratoplasty

PK Test Prausnitz-Kunstner transfer test

PKU phenylketonuria

PL light perception
place
plantar
transpulmonary pressure

PLAP placental alkaline phosphatase

PLBO placebo

PLED periodic lateralizing epileptiform discharge

PLFC premature living female child

PLH paroxysmal localized hyperhidrosis

PLL prolymphocytic leukemia

PLMC premature living male child

PLN pelvic lymph node
popliteal lymph node

PLR pupillary light reflex

PLS plastic surgery

	Preschool Language Scale
	primary lateral sclerosis
PLSO	posterior leafspring orthosis
PLSURG	plastic surgery
PLT	platelet
PLT EST	platelet estimate
plts	platelets
PLV	posterior left ventricular
PM	afternoon
	evening
	pacemaker
	petit mal
	physical medicine
	polymyositis
	poor metabolizers
	post mortem
	presents mainly
	pretibial myxedema
	primary motivation
	prostatic massage
PMA	premenstrual asthma
	Prinzmetal's angina
PMB	polymorphonuclear basophil (leukocytes)
	polymyxin B
	postmenopausal bleeding
PMC	premature mitral closure
	pseudomembranous colitis
PMCP	para-monochlorophenol
PMD	perceptual motor development
	primary myocardial disease
	private medical doctor
PME	polymorphonuclear esosinophil (leukocytes)
	post menopausal estrogen
PMEC	pseudomembranous enterocolitis
PMF	progressive massive fibrosis
PMH	past medical history
PMI	past medical illness
	patient medication instructions
	plea of mental incompetence
	point of maximal impulse
	posterior myocardial infarction
PML	polymorphonuclear leukocytes
	progressive multifocal leukoencephalopathy
PMMF	pectoralis major mycutaneous flat
PMN	polymorphonuclear leukocyte
PMNN	polymorphonuclear neutrophil
PMO	postmenopausal osteoporosis
PMP	pain management program
	previous menstrual period
	psychotropic medication plan
PMPO	postmenopausal palpable ovary
PMR	polymorphic reticulosis
	polymyalgia rheumatica
PM&R	physical medicine and rehabilitation
PMS	postmenopausal syndrome
	post-marketing surveillance
	premenstrual syndrome,
PMT	premenstrual tension
PMTS	premenstrual tension syndrome
PMV	prolapse of mitral valve
PMW	pacemaker wires
PN	parenteral nutrition
	percussion note
	percutaneous nephrostogram
	periarteritis nodosa
	pneumonia
	polynephritis
	poorly nourished
	postnasal
	postnatal
	practical nurse
	premie nipple
	primary nurse
	progress note
P & N	psychiatry and neurology

PNAB	percutaneous needle aspiration biopsy
PNAS	prudent no salt added
PNB	percutaneous needle biopsy
	premature newborn
	premature nodal beat
PNC	penicillin
	peripheral nerve conduction
	premature nodal contraction
	prenatal care
	prenatal course
	Psychiatric Nurse Clinician
PND	paroxysmal nocturnal dyspnea
	pelvic node dissection
	postnasal drip
	pregnancy, not delivered
PNET-MB	primitive neuroectodermal tumors-medulloblastoma
PNF	proprioceptive neuromuscular fasciculation reaction
PNH	paroxysmal nocturnal hemoglobinuria
PNI	peripheral nerve injury
	prognostic nutrition index
PNL	percutaneous nephrostolithotomy
PNMG	persistent neonatal myasthenia gravis
PNP	peak negative pressure
	Pediatric Nurse Practitioner
	progressive nuclear palsey
	purine nucleoside phosphorylase
PNS	partial nonprogressing stroke
	peripheral nervous system
	practical nursing student
PNT	percutaneous nephrostomy tube
pnthx	pneumothorax
PNU	protein nitrogen units
PNV	prenatal vitamins
Pnx	pneumonectomy
	pneumothorax
PO	by mouth (*per os*)
	phone order
	postoperative
PO_2	partial pressure of oxygen
PO_4	phosphate
POA	pancreatic oncofetal antigen
POAG	primary open-angle glaucoma
POB	phenoxybenzamine
	place of birth
POC	postoperative care
	product of conception
POD	pacing on demand
	polycystic ovarian disease
POD 1	postoperative day one
POE	position of ease
POEMS	plasma cell dyscasia with polyneuropathy, organomegaly, endocrinopathy, monoclonal (M)-protein, and skin changes
POF	position of function
P of I	proof of illness
POG	Pediatric Oncology Group
	Penthrane®-oxygen gas (nitrous oxide)
	products of gestation
POHA	preoperative holding area
POHI	physically or otherwise health impaired
POI	Personal Orientation Inventory
POIK	poikilocytosis
POL	premature onset of labor
POLY	polychromic erythrocytes
	polymorphonuclear leukocyte
POLY-CHR	polychromatophilia
POM	pain on motion
	polyoximethylene
	prescription-only medication

POMP	prednisone, vincristine, methotrexate, and mercaptopurine
POMR	problem-oriented medical record
POMS	Profile of Mood States
PONI	postoperative narcotic infusion
POP	pain on palpation persistent occipitoposterior plaster of paris popiliteal
POp	postoperative
poplit	popliteal
POR	problem-oriented record
PORK	porkilocytosis
PORP	partial ossicular replacement prosthesis
PORT	perioperative respiratory therapy postoperative respiratory therapy
POS	parosteal osteosarcoma positive
poss	possible
post	post mortem examination (autopsy)
post op	postoperative
Post Sag D	posterior sagittal diameter
post tib	posterial tibial
POU	placenta, ovaries, and uterus
POW	prisoner of war
PP	near point of accommodation paradoxical pulse partial upper and lower dentures pedal pulse peripheral pulses pin prick plasmapheresis plaster of paris poor person posterior pituitary postpartum postprandial presenting part private patient protoporphyria proximal phalanx pulse pressure push pills
P&P	pins and plaster policy and procedure
PPA	palpitation, percussion, and auscultation phenylpropanolamine phenylpyruvic acid postpartum amenorrhea
PP&A	palpation, percussion, and auscultation
PPAS	post-polio atrophy syndrome
PPB	parts per billion positive pressure breathing
PPBE	postpartum breast engorgment
PPBS	post prandial blood sugar
PPC	progressive patient care
PPD	packs per day posterior polymorphous dystrophy postpartum day purified protein derivative (of tuberculin)
P & PD	percussion & postural drainage
PPD-B	purified protein derivative, Battey
PPD-S	purified protein derivative, standard
PPF	plasma protein fraction
PPG	photoplethysmography postprandial glucose
PPGI	psychophysiologic gastrointestinal (reaction)
PPH	postpartum hemorrhage primary pulmonary hypertension
PPHN	persistent pulmonary hypertension of the newborn
PPI	benzylpenicilloylpolysine patient package insert Present Pain Intensity

PPL pars plana lensectomy
PPLO pleuro-pneumonia-like organisms
PPM parts per million
permanent pacemaker
PPMA post-poliomyelitis muscular atrophy
PPMS psychophysiologic musculoskeletal (reaction)
PPN peripheral parenteral nutrition
PPNAD primary pigmented nodular adrenocortical disease
PPNG penicillinase producing *Neisseria gonorrhoeae*
PPO prefered provider organization
PPP pedal pulse present
peripheral pulses palpable
postpartum psychosis
protamine paracoagulation phenomenon
PPPBL peripheral pulses palpable both legs
PPPG post prandial plasma glucose
PPR patient progress record
PPRC Physician Payment Review Commission
PPROM prolonged premature rupture of membranes
PPS peripheral pulmonary stenosis
postpartum sterilization
PPTL postpartum tubal ligation
PPU perforated peptic ulcer
PPV positive predictive value
PPVT Peabody Picture Vocabulary Test
PQ pronator quadratus
PR far point of accommodation
partial remission
patient relations
per rectum
premature
profile
progressive resistance
prolonged remission
Puerto Rican
pulse rate
P & R pelvic and rectal
pulse and respiration
PRA plasma renin activity
PRAT platelet radioactive antiglobulin test
PRBC packed red blood cells
PRC packed red cells
peer review committee
PRCA pure red cell aplasia
PRD polycystic renal disease
PRE passive resistance exercises
progressive resistive exercise
Pred prednisone
preg Pregestimil®
PREMIE premature infant
pre-op before surgery
prep prepare for surgery
preposition
PRERLA pupils round, equal, react to light and accommodation
prev prevent
previous
PRFN percutaneous radio frequency
PRG phleborheogram
PRH past relevant history
preretinal hemorrhage
PRI Pain Rating Index
prim primary
PRIMIP primipara (1st pregnancy)
PRISM Pediatric Risk of Mortality Score
PRL prolactin
PRLA pupils react to light and accommodation
PRM phosphoribomutase
photoreceptor membrane
prematurely ruptured membrane
PRM-SDX pyrimethamine sulfadoxine
PRN as occasion requires
PRO pronation
protein

	prothrombin
prob	probable
PROCTO	procotoscopic
	proctology
prog.	prognathism
	prognosis
	program
	progressive
PROM	passive range of motion
	premature rupture of membranes
ProMACE	prednisone, methotrexate, calcium leucovorin, doxorubicin, cyclophosphamide, and etoposide
Promy	promyelocyte
PRO MYELO	promyelocytes
PRON	pronation
pros	prostate
	prosthesis
prov	provisional
PROVIMI	proteins, vitamins, and minerals
PROX	proximal
PRP	panretinal photocoagulation
	penicllinase-resistant penicllin
	polyribose ribitol phosphate
	progressive rubella panencephalitis
PRPP	5-phosphoribosyl-1-pyrophosphate
PRRE	pupils round regular, and equal
PRSs	positive rolandic spikes
PRTH-C	prothrombin time control
PRV	polycythemia rubra vera
PRVEP	pattern reversal visual evoked potentials
PRW	polymerized ragweed
PRZ	prazepam
PRZF	pyrazofurin
PS	paradoxic sleep
	paranoid schizophrenia
	pathologic stage
	performance status
	peripheral smear
	plastic surgery (surgeon)
	pressure support
	protective services
	pulmonary stenosis
	pyloricstenosis
	serum from pregnant women
P/S	polyunsaturated to saturated fatty acids ratio
P & S	pain and suffering
	paracentesis and suction
PsA	psoriatic arthritis
PS I	healthy patient with localized pathological process
PS II	a patient with mild to moderate systemic disease
PS III	a patient with severe systemic disease limiting activity but not incapacitating
PS IV	a patient with incapacitating systemic disease
PS V	Moribund patient not expected to live.
	(These are American Society of Anesthesiologists' physical status patient classifications. Emergency operations are designated by "E" after the classification).
PSA	product selection allowed
	prostate-specific antigen
PsA	psoriatic arthritis
PSC	Pediatric Symptom Checklist
	posterior subcapsular cataract
	primary sclerosing cholangitis
PSCT	peripheral stem cell transplant
PSE	portal systemic encephalopathy

PSF	posterior spinal fusion
PSGN	post streptococcal glomerulonephritis
PSH	past surgical history
	post spinal headache
PSI	Physiologic Stability Index
	pounds per square inch
PSIS	posterior superior iliac spine
PSM	presystolic murmur
P/sore	pressure sore
PSP	pancreatic spasmolytic peptide
	phenolsulphthalein
	progressive supranuclear palsy
PSRBOW	premature spontaneous rupture of bag of waters
PSS	painful shoulder syndrome
	physiologic saline solution (0.9% sodium chloride)
	progressive systemic sclerosis
PST	paroxysmal supraventricular tachycardia
	platelet survival time
PSV	pressure supported ventilation
PSVT	paroxysmal supraventricular tachycardia
PSW	psychiatric social worker
PT	cisplatin
	parathormone
	parathyroid
	paroxysmal tachycardia
	patient
	phenytoin
	phototoxicity
	physical therapy
	pine tar
	pint
	posteriortibial
	preterm
	prothrombin time
P&T	paracentesis and tubing (of ears)
	peak and trough
	permanent and total
PTA	percutaneous transluminal angioplasty
	Physical Therapy Assistant
	plasma thromboplastin antecedent
	post-traumatic amnesia
	pretreatment anxiety
	prior to admission
	pure-tone average
PTB	patellar tendon bearing
	prior to birth
	pulmonary tuberculosis
PTBA	percutaneous transluminal balloon angioplasty
PTBD-EF	percutaneous transhepatic biliary drainage—enteric feeding
PTBS	posttraumatic brain syndrome
PTB-SC-SP	patellar tendon bearing-supracondylar-suprapatellar
PTC	patient to call
	percutaneous transhepatic cholangiography
	plasma thromboplastin components
	prior to conception
PT-C	prothrombin time control
PTCA	percutaneous transluminal coronary angioplasty
PTCL	peripheral T-cell lymphoma
PTCR	percutaneous transluminal coronary recanalization
PTD	period to discharge
	permanent and total disability
	prior to delivery
PTDP	permanent transvenous demand pacemaker
PTE	pretibial edema
	proximal tibial epiphysis
	pulmonary thromboembolism
PTED	pulmonary thromboembolic disease

PTFE polytetrafluorethylene
PTG parathyroid gland
teniposide
PTH parathyroid hormone
post transfusion hepatitis
prior to hospitalization
PTHC percutaneous transhepatic cholangiography
PTJV percutaneous transtracheal jet ventilation
PTL pre-term labor
Sodium Pentothal®
PTMDF pupils, tension, media, disc, and fundus
PTNM postsurgical resection-pathologic staging of cancer
PTO please turn over
PTP posterior tibial pulse
PTPM posttraumatic progressive myelopathy
PTPN peripheral (vein) total parenteral nutrition
PTR patella tendon reflex
patient to return
prothrombin time ratio
PT-R prothrombin time ratio
PTS patellar tendon suspension
permanent threshold shift
prior to surgery
PTSD post-traumatic stress disorder
PTT partial thromboplastin time
platelet transfusion therapy
PTT-C partial thromboplastin time control
PTU pain treatment unit
propylthiouracil
PTV posterior tibial vein
PTWTKG patient's weight in kilograms
PTX parathyroidectomy
pelvic traction
pneumothorax
PTZ pentylenetetrazol
phenothiazine
PU pelvic-ureteric
peptic ulcer
pregnancy urine
PUBS percutaneous umbilical blood sampling
PUD peptic ulcer disease
PUE pyrexia of unknown etiology
PUFA polyunsaturated fatty acids
pul. pulmonary
PUN plasma urea nitrogen
PUO pyrexia of unknown origin
PUP percutaneous ultrasonic pyelolithotomy
PUPP pruritic urticarial papules and plaque of pregnancy
PUVA psoralen-ultraviolet-light (treatment)
PV papillomavirus
per vagina
polio vaccine
polycythemia vera
popliteal vein
portal vein
postvoiding
pulmonary vein
P&V peak and valley (this is a dangerous abbreviation) use peak and trough
pyloroplasty and vagotomy
PVA polyvinyl alcohol
Prinzmental's variant angina
PVB cisplatin, vinblastine, and bleomycin
premature ventricular beat
PVC polyvinyl chloride
postvoiding cystogram
premature ventricular contraction
pulmonary venous congestion
PVD patient very disturbed
peripheral vascular disease
posterior vitreous detachment

	premature ventricular depolarization
PVE	perivenous encephalomyelitis
	premature ventricular extrasystole
	prosthetic value endocarditis
PVF	peripheral visual field
PVFS	postviral fatigue syndrome
PVH	periventricular hemorrhage
	pulmonary vascular hypertension
PVI	peripheral vascular insufficiency
PVK	penicillin V potassium
PVM	proteins, vitamins, and minerals
PVNS	pigmented villonodular synovitis
PVO	peripheral vascular occlusion
	pulmonary venous occlusion
PVO_2	mixed venous pressure of oxygen
PVOD	pulmonary vascular obstructive disease
PVP	cisplatin and etoposide
	peripheral venous pressure
	polyvinylpyrrolidone
P-VP-B	cisplatin, etoposide, and bleomycin
PVR	peripheral vascular resistance
	postvoiding residual
	proliferative vitreoretinopathy
	pulmonary vascular resistance
	pulse-volume recording
PVS	percussion, vibration and suction
	peritoneovenous shunt
	persistent vegetative state
	Plummer-Vinson syndrome
	pulmonic valve stenosis
PVT	paroxysmal ventricular tachycardia
	private
PW	pacing wires
	patient waiting
	puncture wound
P&W	pressures and waves
PWB	partial weight bearing
	psychological well-being
PWI	pediatric walk-in clinic
	posterior wall infarct
PWLV	posterior wall of left ventricle
PWM	pokeweed mitogens
PWP	pulmonary wedge pressure
PWS	port-wine stain
PWV	polistes wasp venom
Px	physical exam
	pneumothorax
	prognosis
PXE	pseudoxanthoma elasticum
PY	pack years
PYP	pyrophosphate
PZ	peripheral zone
PZA	pyrazinamide
PZI	protamine zinc insulin

Q

q	every
QA	quality assurance
QAM	every morning (this is a dangerous abbreviation)
QC	quality control
	quick catheter
QCA	quantitative coronary angiography
qd	every day (this is a dangerous abbreviation as it is read as four times daily)
q4h	every four hours
qh	every hour
qhs	every night (this is a dangerous abbreviation as it is read as every hour)

qid four times daily
QIG quantitative immunoglobulins
QMI Q wave myocardial infarction
QMRP qualified mental retardation professional
QMT quantitative muscle testing
q.n. every night (this is a dangerous abbreviation as it is read as every hour)
q.n.s. quantity not sufficient
qod every other day (this is a dangerous abbreviation as it is read as every day or four times a day)
qoh every other hour (this is a dangerous abbreviation as it is read as every day or four times a day)
QON every other night (this is a dangerous abbreviation)
qpm every evening (this is a dangerous abbreviation)
QR quiet room
QRS principal deflection in an electrocardiogram
Q.S. every shift
sufficient quantity
Qs/Qt intrapulmonary shunt fraction
QSP physiological shunt fraction
qt quart
QTC quantitative tip cultures
QUAD quadrant
quadriceps
quadriplegic
QU quiet
QUART quadrantectomy, axillary dissection, and radiotherapy
qwk once a week (this is a dangerous abbreviation)

R

R rate
rectal
rectum
regular
regular insulin
resistant
respiration
right
roentgen
Ⓡ right
RA rales
repeat action
retinoic acid
rheumatoid arthritis
right arm
right atrium
right auricle
room air
RAA renin-angiotensin-aldosterone
RAAS renin-angiotensin-aldosterone system
RABG room air blood gas
RAC right atrial catheter
RACCO right anterior caudocranial oblique
RACT recalcified whole-blood activated clotting time
RAD ionizing radiation unit
radical
radiology
reactive airway disease
right axis deviation
RAE right atrial enlargement
RAEB refractory anemia, erythroblastic
RAG room air gas
RAH right atrial hypertrophy
RAIU radioactive iodine uptake
RALT routine admission laboratory tests
RAM radioactive material
rapid alternating movements
RAN resident's admission notes
R_2AN second year resident's admission notes

RAO right anterior oblique
RAP right atrial pressure
RAQ right anterior quadrant
RAPD relative afferent pupillary defect
RAS renal artery stenosis
RAST radioallergosorbent test
RAT right anterior thigh
RA test test for rheumatoid factor
RATx radiation therapy
R(AW) airway resistance
RB retinoblastoma
retrobulbar
right buttock
R & B right and below
RBA right basilar artery
right brachial artery
RBB right breast biopsy
RBBB right bundle branch block
RBBX right breast biopsy examination
RBC red blood cell (count)
RBCD right border cardiac dullness
RBCM red blood cell mass
RBC s/f red blood cells spun filtration
RBCV red blood cell volume
RBD right border of dullness
RBE relative biologic effectiveness
RBF renal blood flow
RBG random blood glucose
RBOW rupture bag of water
RBP retinol-binding protein
RBS random blood sugar
RBV right brachial vein
RC Red Cross
Roman Catholic
rotator cuff
R/C reclining chair
RCA radionuclide cerebral angiogram
right coronary artery
RCBF regional cerebral blood flow
RCC renal cell carcinoma
RCCT randomized controlled clinical trial
RCD relative cardiac dullness
RCF Reiter complement fixation
RCHF right-sided congestive heart failure
RCM radiographic contrast media
retinal capillary microaneurysm
right costal margin
RCPM raven coloured progressive matrices
RCPT Registered Cardiopulmonary Technician
RCS repeat cesarean section
reticulum cell sarcoma
RCT randomized clinical trial
Registered Care Technologist
root canal therapy
Rorschach Content Test
RCV red cell volume
R.D. Registered Dietitian
RD Raynaud's disease
reflex decay
renal disease
respiratory disease
retinal detachment
Reye's disease
right deltoid
ruptured disc
RDA recommended daily allowance
RDG right dorsogluteal
RDH Registered Dental Hygienist
RDIH right direct inguinal hernia
RDOD retinal detachment, right eye
RDOS retinal detachment, left eye
RDP right dorsoposterior
RDPE reticular degeneration of the pigment epithelium
RDS research diagnostic criteria
respiratory distress syndrome

RDT	regular dialysis (hemodialysis) treatment
RDTD	referral, diagnosis, treatment, and discharge
RDVT	recurrent deep vein thrombosis
RDW	red (cell) distribution width
RE	concerning
	rectal examination
	reflux esophagitis
	regional enteritis
	reticuloendothelial
	retinol equivalents
	right ear
	right eye
R & E	rest and exercise
	round and equal
R↑E	right upper extremity
RE ✓	recheck
REC	rear end collision
	recommend
	record
	recovery
	recreation
	recur
RECT	rectum
RED SUBS	reducing substances
REE	resting energy expenditure
R-EEG	resting electroencephalogram
REF	referred
	refused
	renal erythropoietic factor
ref →	refer to
Reg block	regional block anesthesia
regurg	regurgitation
rehab	rehabilitation
REL	relative
	religion
REM	rapid eye movement
	recent event memory
REMS	rapid eye movement sleep
REP	repair
	repeat
	report
repol	repolarization
REPS	repetitions
RER	renal excretion rate
RES	resection
	resident
	reticuloendothelial system
RESC	resuscitation
resp.	respirations
	respiratory
REST	restoration
RET	retention
	reticulocyte
	retina
	retired
	return
	right esotropia
retic	reticulocyte
REV	reverse
	review
	revolutions
RF	renal failure
	rheumatic fever
	rheumatoid factor
	risk factor
R&F	radiographic and fluoroscopic
RFA	right femoral artery
	right fronto-anterior
RFL	right frontolateral
RFLP	restriction fragment length polymorphism
RFM	rifampin
RFP	request for payment
	right frontoposterior
RFS	rapid frozen section
RFT	right frontotransverse
	routine fever therapy
RG	right gluteal
RGM	right gluteus medius
RGO	reciprocating gait orthosis
Rh	Rhesus factor in blood
RH	reduced haloperidol
	rest home
	retinal hemorrhage
	right hand
	right hyperphoria
	room humidifier
RHB	raise head of bed
RHC	respiration has ceased
RHD	relative hepatic dullness
	rheumatic heart disease

RHF	right heart failure
RHG	right hand grip
RHH	right homonymous hemianopsia
RHL	right hemisphere lesions
rHmEPO	recombinant human erythropoietin
RHS	right hand side
RHT	right hypertropia
RHW	radiant heat warmer
RI	regular insulin
	rooming in
RIA	radioimmunoassay
RIAT	radioimmune antiglobulin test
RIC	right iliac crest
	right internal carotid (artery)
RICE	rest, ice, compression, and elevation
RICM	right intercostal margin
RICS	right intercostal space
RICU	respiratory intensive care unit
RID	radial immunodiffusion
	ruptured intervertebral disc
RIE	rocket immunoelectrophoresis
RIF	rifampin
	right iliac fossa
	right index finger
	rigid internal fixation
RIG	rabies immune globulin
RIH	right inguinal hernia
RIMA	right internal mammary anastamosis
RIND	reversible ischemic neurologic defect
RIP	radioimmunoprecipitin test
	rapid infusion pump
RIR	right inferior rectus
RISA	radioactive iodinated serum albumin
RIST	radioimmunosorbent test
RK	radial keratotomy
	right kidney
RL	right lateral
	right leg
	right lung
	Ringer's lactate
R→L	right to left
RLBCD	right lower border of cardiac dullness
RLC	residual lung capacity
RLD	related living donor
	right later decubitus
RLE	right lower extremity
RLF	retrolental fibroplasia
RLL	right lower lobe
RLN	recurrent laryngeal nerve
RLQ	right lower quadrant
RLR	right lateral rectus
RLS	Ringer's lactate solution
RLT	right lateral thigh
RLTCS	repeat low transverse cesarean section
RM	radical mastectomy
	repetitions maximum
	respiratory movement
	room
R&M	routine and microscopic
RMA	right mento-anterior
RMCA	right main coronary artery
	right middle cerebral artery
RMCL	right midclavicular line
RMD	rapid movement disorder
RME	resting metabolic expenditure
	right mediolateral episiotomy
RMEE	right middle ear exploration
RMK #1	remark number 1
RML	right mediolateral
	right middle lobe
RMLE	right mediolateral episiotomy
RMP	right mentoposterior
RMR	resting metabolic rate
	right medial rectus
RMS	repetitive motion syndrome
RMS®	Rectal Morphine Sulfate (suppository)
RMSE	root mean square error
RMSF	Rocky Mountain spotted fever

RMT	Registered Music Therapist
	right mentotransverse
RN	Registered Nurse
RNA	radionuclide angiography
	ribonucleic acid
RND	radical neck dissection
RNEF	resting (radio-) nuclide ejection fraction
RO	routine order
R/O	rule out
ROA	right occiput anterior
ROAC	repeated oral doses of activated charcoal
ROC	receiver operating characteristic
	resident on call
	residual organic carbon
ROI	region of interest
ROIDS	hemorrhoids
ROIH	right oblique inguinal hernia
ROL	right occipitolateral
ROM	range of motion
	right otitis media
	rupture of membranes
Romb	Romberg
ROMSA	right otitis media, suppurative, acute
ROMSC	right otitis media, suppurative, chronic
ROP	retinopathy of prematurity
	right occiput posterior
RoRx	radiation therapy
ROS	review of systems
	rod outer segments
ROSC	restoration of spontaneous circulation
ROT	remedial occupational therapy
	right occipital transverse
	rotator
ROUL	rouleaux
RP	radial pulse
	radiopharmaceutical
	Raynaud's phenomenon
	retinitis pigmentosa
	retrograde pyelogram
RPA	radial photon absorptiometry
	Registered Physician's Assistant
	right pulmonary artery
RPCF	Reiter protein complement fixation
RPD	removable partial denture
RPE	rating of perceived exertion
	retinal pigment epithelium
RPF	relaxed pelvic floor
	renal plasma flow
RPG	retrograde pyelogram
RPGN	rapidly progressive glomerulonephritis
RPH	retroperitoneal hemorrhage
R.Ph.	Registered Pharmacist
RPHA	reverse passive hemagglutination
RPICCE	round pupil intracapsular cataract extraction
RPL	retroperitoneal lymphadenectomy
RPN	renal papillary necrosis
	resident's progress notes
R_2PN	second year resident's progress notes
RPO	right posterior oblique
RPP	rate-pressure product
RPR	rapid plasma reagin (test for syphilis)
	Reiter protein reagin
RPT	Registered Physical Therapist
RPTA	Registered Physical Therapist Assistant
RQ	respiratory quotient
RR	recovery room
	regular respirations
	respiratory rate
	retinal reflex
R/R	rales-rhonchi
R&R	rate and rhythm
	recent and remote
	recession and resection
	rest and recuperation
RRA	radioreceptor assay
	Registered Record Administrator

RRAM	rapid rhythmic alternating movements
RRCT, no(m)	regular rate, clear tones, no murmurs
RRE	round, regular, and equal (pupils)
RREF	resting radionuclide ejection fraction
rRNA	ribosomal ribonucleic acid
RRND	right radical neck dissection
RROM	resistive range of motion
RRR	regular rhythm and rate
RRRN	round, regular, and react normally
RRT	Registered Respiratory Therapist
RS	Raynaud's syndrome
	Reiter's syndrome
	Reye's syndrome
	rhythm strip
	right side
	Ringer's solution
R/S	rest stress
	rupture spontaneous
RSA	right sacrum anterior
	right subclavian artery
RScA	right scapuloanterior
RScP	right scapuloposterior
rscu-PA	recombinant, single-chain, urokinase-type plasminogen activator
RSDS	reflex-sympathetic dystrophy syndrome
R-SICU	respiratory-surgical intensive care unit
RSO	right salpingo-oophorectomy
	right superior oblique
RSP	right sacroposterior
RSR	regular sinus rhythm
	relative survival rate
	right superior rectus
RSS	Russian spring-summer (encephalitis)
RST	right sacrum transverse
RSTs	Rodney Smith tubes
RSV	respiratory syncytial virus
	right subclavian vein
RSW	right-sided weakness
RT	radiation therapy
	recreational therapy
	rectal temperature
	renal transplant
	repetition time
	respiratory therapist
	right
	right thigh
	running total
R/t	related to
RTA	renal tubular acidosis
RTC	return to clinic
	round the clock
RTER	return to emergency room
rt. ↑ ext.	right upper extremity
RTF	return to flow
RTL	reactive to light
RTM	routine medical care
RTN	renal tubular necrosis
RTNM	retreatment staging of cancer
RTO	return to office
RTOG	Radiation Therapy Oncology Group
rtPA	recombinant tissue-type plasminogen
RTRR	return to recovery room
RTS	real time scan
	return to sender
RT_3U	resin triiodothyronine uptake
RTUS	realtime ultrasound
RTW	return to work
RTWD	return to work determination
RTx	radiation therapy
RU	routine urinalysis
RUA	routine urine analysis
RUE	right upper extremity
RUG	retrograde urethrogram
RUL	right upper lobe
RUOQ	right upper outer quadrant
rupt.	ruptured
RUQ	right upper quadrant
RURTI	recurrent upper respiratory tract infection
RUSB	right upper sternal border
RV	rectovaginal

	residual volume
	respiratory volume
	return visit
	right ventricle
	rubella vaccine
RVAD	right ventricular assist device
RVD	relative vertebral density
RVE	right ventricular enlargement
RVEDP	right ventricular end-diastolic pressure
RVET	right ventricular ejection time
RVF	Rift-Valley fever
	right ventricular function
RVG	radionuclide ventriculography
	right ventrogluteal
RVH	right ventricular hypertrophy
RVIDd	right ventricle internal dimension diastole
RVL	right vastus lateralis
RVO	relaxed vaginal outlet
	retinal vein occlusion
	right ventricular outflow
	right ventricular overactivity
RVOT	right ventricular outflow tract
RVR	rapid ventricular response
RVP	right ventricular pressure
RVS	rabies vaccine, adsorbed
RVSWI	right ventricular stroke work index
RVT	renal vein thrombosis
RV/TLC	residual volume to total lung capacity ratio
RVV	rubella vaccine virus
RVVT	Russell's viper venom time
RW	ragweed
R/W	return to work
RWM	regional wall motion
Rx	drug
	medication
	pharmacy
	prescription
	radiotherapy
	take
	therapy
	treatment
RXN	reaction
RXT	radiation therapy
	right exotropia

S

S	sacral
	second (s)
	semilente insulin
	sensitive
	serum
	single
	sister
	son
	subjective findings
	suction
	sulfur
	supervision
$\bar{s}$	without (this is a dangerous abbreviation)
S_1	first heart sound
S_2	second heart sound
S_3	third heart sound (ventricular gallop)
S_4	fourth hear sound (atrial gallup)
$S_1 \ldots S_5$	sacral vertebra 1 through 5
SA	salicylic acid
	sleep apnea
	sinoatrial
	sinoatrial
	Spanish American
	suicide alert
	suicide attempt
	surface area
	surgical assistant
	sustained action
S/A	same as
	sugar and acetone
S&A	sugar and acetone
SAA	same as above
SAB	serum albumin
	spontaneous abortion
	subarachnoid bleed
	subarachnoid block

SAC — short arm cast; substance abuse counselor
SACC — short arm cylinder cast
SACH — solid ankle cushion heel
SAD — seasonal affective disorder; Self-Assessment Depression (scale); subacute dialysis; sugar and acetone determination
SADL — simulated activities of daily living
SADR — suspected adverse drug reaction
SADS — Schedule for Affective Disorders and Schizophrenia
SAE — short above elbow (cast)
SAF — self-articulating femoral
Sag D — sagittal diameter
SAH — subarachnoid hemorrhage; systemic arterial hypertension
SAI — Sodium Amytal interview
SAL — salicylate; *Salmonella*
SAL 12 — sequential analysis of 12 chemistry constituents
SAM — self-administered medication; systolic anterior motion
SAN — side-arm nebulizer; sinoatrial node; slept all night
SANC — short arm navicular cast
sang — sanguinous
SAO — small airway obstruction
SaO_2 — arterial oxygen percent saturation
SAPD — self administration of psychotropic drugs
SAPH — saphenous
SAPS — short arm plaster splint; Simplified Acute Physiology Score
SAQ — short arc quad
SAR — seasonal allergic rhinitis; sexual attitudes reassessment
SARA — sexually acquired reactive arthritis; system for anesthetic and respiratory administration
SAS — saline, agent, and saline; self-rating anxiety scale; short arm splint; sleep apnea syndrome; subarachnoid space; sulfasalazine
SASH — saline, agent, saline, and heparin
SAT — saturated; saturation; Saturday; speech awareness threshold; subacute thyroiditis
SATL — surgical Achilles tendon lengthening
SAVD — spontaneous assisted vaginal delivery
SB — safety belt; sandbag; Sengstaken-Blakemore (tube); sinus bradycardia; small bowel; spina bifida; stand-by; Stanford-Binet; sternal border; stillbirth; stillborn
Sb — antimony
S/B — side bending
SBA — serum bactericidal activity; standby assistant (assistance)
SBC — standard bicarbonate; strict bed confinement
SBE — short below elbow (cast); shortness of breath on exertion; subacute bacterial endocarditis
SBFT — small bowel follow through
SBG — stand-by guard

SBGM self blood glucose monitoring
SBI systemic bacterial infection
SB-LM Stanford Binet Intelligence Test-Form LM
SBO small bowel obstruction
SBOD scleral buckle, right eye
SBOH State Board of Health
SBOM soybean oil meal
SBOS scleral buckle, left eye
SBP school breakfast program
scleral buckling procedure
small bowel phytobezoars
spontaneous bacterial peritonitis
systolic blood pressure
SBQC small based quad cane
SBR strict bed rest
SBS shaken baby syndrome
short bowel syndrome
SBT serum bactericidal titers
SBTT small bowel transit time
SC schizophrenia
self-care
serum creatinine
service connected
sickle-cell
Snellen's chart
spinal cord
sternoclavicular
subclavian
subclavian
subcutaneous
sulfur colloid
without correction (without glasses)
SCA subcutaneous abdominal (block)
SCAN suspected child abuse and neglect
SCAT sheep cell agglutination titer
sickle cell anemia test
SCB strictly confined to bed
SCBC small cell bronchogenic carcinoma
SCBF spinal cord blood flow
SCC sickle cell crisis
squamous cell carcinoma
SCCa squamous cell carcinoma
SCCA semi-closed circle absorber
SCD sequential compression device
service connected disability
sickle cell disease
spinal cord disease
subacute combined degeneration
sudden cardiac death
ScDA scapulodextra anterior
ScDP scapulodextra posterior
SCE sister chromatid exchange
SCEMIA self-contained enzymic membrane immunoassay
SCEP somatosensory cortical evoked potential
SCFE slipped capitol femoral epiphysis
SCG sodium cromoglycate
SCh succinylcholine chloride
SCHISTO schistocytes
SCHIZ schizocytes
schizophrenia
SCHLP supracricord hemilaryngopharyngectomy
SCI spinal cord injury
SCID severe combined immunodeficiency disorders
SCIPP sacrococcygeal to inferior pubic point
SCIU spinal cord injury unit
SCIV subclavian intravenous
SCL skin conductance level
symptom checklist
SCL-90 symptoms checklist—90 items
ScLA scapulolaeva anterior
SCLC small-cell lung cancer
SCLE subcutaneous lupus erythematosis
ScLP scapulolaeva posterior

SCLs	soft contact lenses
SCM	sensation, circulation, and motion
	spondylitic caudal myelopathy
	sternocleidomastoid
SCMD	senile choroidal macular degeneration
SCN	special care nursery
SCOP	scopolamine
SCP	sodium cellulose phosphate
SCR	special care room (seclusion room)
	spondylitic caudal radioculopathy
SCr	serum creatinine
SCT	sickel cell trait
	sugar coated tablet
SCU	self-care unit
	special care unit
SCUF	slow and continuous ultrafiltration
SCUT	schizophrenia chronic undifferentiated type
SCV	subclavian vein
	subcutaneous vaginal (block)
SD	scleroderma
	senile dementia
	septal defect
	severely disabled
	shoulder disarticulation
	spontaneous delivery
	standard deviation
	standard diet
	sterile dressing
	straight drainage
	streptozocin and doxorubicin
	sudden death
	surgical drain
S & D	stomach and duodenum
SDA	sacrodextra anterior
	Seventh-Day Adventist
	steroid-dependent asthmatic
SDAT	senile dementia of Alzheimer's type
SDB	sleep disordered breathing
SDC	serum digoxin concentration
	sodium deoxycholate
SD&C	suction, dilation, and curettage
SDB	self-destructive behavior
SDC	sleep disorders center
SDD	selective digestive (tract) decontamination
SDH	subdural hematoma
SDL	serum digoxin level
	serum drug level
	speech discrimination loss
SDP	sacrodextra posterior
	stomach, duodenum, and pancreas
SDS	same day surgery
	Self-Rating Depression Scale
SDT	sacrodextra transversa
	speech detection threshold
SDU	step-down unit
SE	saline enema
	side effect
	soft exudates
	spin echo
	standard error
	Starr-Edwards
Se	selenium
sec	second
	secondary
	secretary
SECPR	standard external cardiopulmonary resuscitation
SED	sedimentation
	spondyloepiphyseal dysplasia
sed rt	sedimentation rate
SEER	Surveillance, Epidemiology, and End Results (program)
SEG	segment
seg	segmented neutrophils
SEH	subependymal hemorrhage
SEI	subepithelial (corneal) infiltrate

SELFVD	sterile elective low forceps vaginal delivery
SEM	scanning electron microscopy
	semen
	standard error of mean
	systolic ejection murmur
SEMI	subendocardial myocardial infarction
SENS	sensitivity
	sensorium
SEP	separate
	somatosensory evoked potential
	systolic ejection period
SEQ	sequella
SER	scanning equalization radiography
SER-IV	supination external rotation, type 4 fracture
SERs	somatosensory evoked responses
SES	socioeconomic status
SEWHO	shoulder-elbow-wrist-hand orthosis
SF	salt free
	saturated fat
	scarlet fever
	seizure frequency
	seminal fluid
	soft feces
	spinal fluid
	sugar free
	symptom-free
	synovial fluid
S&F	soft and flat
SFA	saturated fatty acids
	superficial femoral artery
SFC	spinal fluid count
SFEMG	single-fiber electromyography
SFP	spinal fluid pressure
SFPT	standard fixation preference test
SFTR	sagittal, frontal, transverse, rotation
SFV	superficial femoral vein
SG	salivary gland
	serum glucose
	skin graft
	specific gravity
	Swan-Ganz
SGA	small for gestational age
SGC	Swan-Ganz catheter
SGD	straight gravity drainage
SGE	significant glandular enlargement
$\bar{s}$ gl	without correction/without glasses
SGOT	serum glutamic oxaloacetic transaminase (same as AST)
SGPT	serum glutamic pyruvic transaminase (same as ALT)
SGS	second generation sulfonylurea
	subglottic stenosis
SH	serum hepatitis
	short
	shoulder
	shower
	social history
	surgical history
S&H	speech and hearing
S/H	suicidal/homicidal ideation
SHA	super heated aerosol
S Hb	sickle hemoglobin screen
SHEENT	skin, head, eyes, ears, nose, and throat
Shig	*Shigella*
SHL	supraglottic horizontal laryngectomy
SHS	student health service
SI	International System of Units
	sacroiliac
	self-inflicted
	seriously ill
	small intestine
	strict isolation
	stress incontinence
	stroke index
SIADH	syndrome of inappropriate antidiuretic hormone secretion
S & I	suction and irrigation
SIB	self-injurious behavior

sibs	siblings
SICT	selective intracoronary thrombolysis
SICU	surgical intensive care unit
SIDS	sudden infant death syndrome
Sig.	let it be marked (appears on prescription before directions for patient)
SIJ	sacroiliac joint
SILFVD	sterile indicated low forceps vaginal delivery
SIM	selective ion monitoring Similac®
Sim c̄ Fe	Similac with iron®
SIMV	synchronized intermittent mandatory ventilation
SIS	sister
SISI	short increment sensitivity index
SIT	Slossen Intelligence Test sperm immobilization test
SIT BAL	sitting balance
SIT TOL	sitting tolerance
SIV	Simian immunodeficiency virus
SIW	self-inflicted wound
SJS	Stevens-Johnson syndrome Swyer-James syndrome
SK	senile keratosis SmithKline® solar keratosis streptokinase
SK 65®	propoxyphene HCl 65 mg
SKAO	supracondylar knee-ankle orthosis
SK-SD	streptokinase streptodornase
SL	sensation level shortleg slight sublingual
S/L	slit lamp (examination)
SLA	sacrolaeva anterior slide latex agglutination
SLB	short leg brace
SLC	short leg cast
SLCC	short leg cylinder cast
SLE	slit lamp examination systemic lupus erythematosus
SLFVD	sterile low forceps vaginal delivery
SLGXT	symptom limited graded exercise test
SLK	superior limbic keratoconjunctivitis
SLMFVD	sterile low mid-forceps vaginal delivery
SLMP	since last menstrual period
SLN	superior laryngeal nerve
SLNTG	sublingual nitroglycerin
SLNWBC	short leg nonweight-bearing cast
SLNWC	short leg non-walking cast
SLO	streptolysin O
SLR	straight leg raising
SLRT	straight leg raising test
SLS	short leg splint single limb support
SLT	swing light test
SLT	sacrolaeva transversa
sl. tr.	slight trace
SLUD	salivation, lacrimation, urination, and defecation
SLWC	short leg walking cast
SM	sadomasochism skim milk small streptomycin systolic murmur
SMA	sequential multiple analyzer simultaneous multichannel auto-analyzer spinal muscular atrophy superior mesenteric artery
SMA-6	sequential multipler analyzer for sodium, potassium, CO_2, chloride, glucose, and BUN
SMA-7	sodium, potassium, CO_2, chloride, glucose, BUN, and creatinine

SMA-12 glucose, BUN, uric acid, calcium, phosphorus, total protein, albumin, cholesterol, total bilirubin, alkaline phosphatase, SGOT, and LDH
SMA-23 includes the entire SMA-12 plus sodium, potassium, CO_2, chloride, direct bilirubin, triglyceride, SGPT, indirect bilirubin, R fraction, and BUN/creatinine ratio
SMAS superficial musculoaponeurotic system
SMBG self-monitoring blood glucose
SMC special mouth care
SMCD senile macular chorioretinal degeneration
SMD senile macular degeneration
SMF streptozocin, mitomycin, and fluorouracil
SMFVD sterile mid-forceps vaginal delivery
SMI sensory motor integration (group)
severely mentally impaired
small volume infusion
sustained maximal inspiration
safety, monitoring, intervention, length of stay and evaluation
SMILE sustained maximal inspiratory lung exercises
SMO Senior Medical Officer
slip made out
SMON subacute myeloopticoneuropathy
SMP self-management program
SMR senior medical resident
skeletal muscle relaxant
standardized mortality ratio
submucosal resection
SMRR submucous resection and rhinoplasty
SMS senior medical student
somatostatin
SMV submentovertical
superior mesenteric vein
SMVT sustained monomorphic ventricular tachycardia
SN sciatic notch
student nurse
Sn tin
S/N signal to noise ratio
SNA specimen not available
SNAP sensory nerve action potential
SNB scalene node biopsy
SNC skilled nursing care
SNCV sensory nerve conduction velocity
SND single needle device
sinus node dysfunction
SNE subacute necrotizing encephalomyelopathy
SNF skilled nursing facility
SNGFR single nephron glomerular filtration rate
SNHL sensorineural hearing loss
SNOOP Systematic Nursing Observation of Psychopathology
SNP sodium nitroprusside
SNS sterile normal saline (0.9% sodium chloride)
SNT sinuses, nose, and throat
suppan nail technique
SO second opinion
shoulder orthosis
significant other
sphincter of Oddi
standing orders
suboccipital
superior oblique
supraoptic
supraorbital
sutures out
S-O salpingo-oophorectomy
S&O salpingo-oophorectomy

SO_3	sulfite
SO_4	sulfate
SOA	serum opsonic activity
	spinal opioid analgesia
	supraorbital artery
	swelling of ankles
SOAA	signed out against advice
SOAM	sutures out in the morning
SOAMA	signed out against medical advice
SOAP	subjective, objective, assessment, and plans
SOAPIE	subjective, objective, assessment, plan, intervention, and evaluation
SOB	shortness of breath (this abbreviation has caused problems)
	see order book
	side of bed
SOC	socialization
	standard of care
S & OC	signed and on chart (e.g. permit)
SOD	sinovenous occlusive disease
	superoxide dysmutase
	surgical officer of the day
SOG	suggestive of good
SOL	solution
	space occupying lesion
SOM	serous otitis media
SOMI	sterno-occipital mandibular immobilizer
Sono	sonogram
SONP	solid organs not palpable
SOP	standard operating procedure
SOPM	stitches out in afternoon
SOR	sign own release
SOS	may be repeated once if urgently required (Latin: *si opus sit*)
	self-obtained smear
SOT	something other than
	stream of thought
SP	sacrum to pubis
	semiprivate
	sequential pulse
	speech
	spouse
	stand pivot
	suicide precautions
	suprapubic
sp	species
S/P	semiprivate
	serum protein
	spinal
	stand and pivot
	status post
	suicide precautions
	suprapubic
	systolic pressure
SPA	albumin human (formerly known as salt-poor albumin)
	serum prothrombin activity
	stimulation produced analgesia
SPAG	small particle aerosol generator
SPAMM	spatial modulation of magnetization
SPBI	serum protein bound iodine
SPBT	suprapubic bladder tap
SPD	subcorneal pustular dermatosis
SPET	single-photon emission tomography
SPE	serum protein electrophoresis
SPEC	specimen
SPECT	single photon emission computer tomography
Spec Ed	special education
SPEP	serum protein electrophoresis
SPET	single-photon emission tomography
SPF	split products of fibrin
	sun protective factor
sp fl	spinal fluid
SPG	sphenopalatine ganglion
Sp.G.	specific gravity
SPH	spherocytes
SPHERO	spherocytes
SPI	speech processor interface

SPIA	solid phase immunoabsorbent assay
SPIF	spontaneous peak inspiratory force
SPL	sound pressure level
SPK	superficial punctate keratitis
SPMA	spinal progressive muscle atrophy
SPN	solitary pulmonary nodule
	student practical nurse
spont	spontaneous
SPP	species (specus)
	suprapubic prostatectomy
SPROM	spontaneous premature rupture of membrane
SPS	simple partial seizure
	sodium polyethanol sulfanate
	systemic progressive sclerosis
SPT	skin prick test
SP TAP	spinal tap
SPU	short procedure unit
SPVR	systemic peripheral vascular resistance
SQ	status quo
	subcutaneous (this is a dangerous abbreviation)
Sq CCa	squamous cell carcinoma
SR	screen
	sedimentation rate
	side rails
	sinus rhythm
	smooth-rough
	sustained release
	system review
S&R	seclusion and restraint
SRBC	sheep red blood cells
	sickle red blood cells
SRBOW	spontaneous rupture of bag of waters
SRD	service-related disability
	sodium-restricted diet
SRF	somatotropin releasing factor
	subretinal fluid
SRF-A	slow releasing factor of anaphylaxis
SRH	signs of recent hemorrhage
SRIF	somatotropin-releaseinhibiting factor (Somatostin)
SRMD	stress-related mucosal damage
SR/NE	sinus rhythm, no ectopy
SRNVM	senile retinal neovascular membrane
	subretinal neovascular membrane
SRO	single room occupancy
SROM	spontaneous rupture of membrane
SRP	stapes replacement prosthesis
SRS-A	slow-reacting substance of anaphylaxis
SRT	sedimentation rate test
	speech reception threshold
	sustained release theophylline
SRU	side rails up
SRUS	solitary rectal ulcer syndrome
SS	half
	sacrosciatic
	saline solution
	saliva sample
	salt substitute
	sickle cell
	Sjögren's syndrome
	sliding scale
	slip sent
	Social Security
	social service
	somatostatin
	susceptible
	symmetrical strength
S&S	shower and shampoo
	signs and symptoms
	support & stimulation
SSA	sagittal split advancement
	salicylsalicylic acid (salsalate)
	Sjögren's syndrome antigen A
	Social Security Administration

	sulfasalicylic acid (test)
SSc	systemic sclerosis
SSCA	single shoulder contrast arthrography
SSCP	substernal chest pain
SSCr	stainless steel crown
SSCVD	sterile spontaneous controlled vaginal delivery
SSD	sickle cell disease
	silver sulfadiazine
	Social Security disability
	source to skin distance
SSDI	Social Security disability income
SSE	saline solution enema
	soapsuds enema
	systemic side effects
SSEPs	somatosensory evoked potentials
SSF	subscapular skinfold (thickness)
SSG	sublabial salivary gland
SSI	sub-shock insulin
	Supplemental Security Income
SSKI	saturated solution of potassium iodide
SSM	superficial spreading melanoma
SSN	Social Security number
SSO	Spanish speaking only
SSOP	Second Surgical Opinion Program
SSPE	subacute sclerosing panencephalitis
SSPL	saturation sound pressure level
SSPU	surgical short procedure unit
SSS	layer upon layer
	scalded skin syndrome
	sick sinus syndrome
	sterile saline soak
SSSB	sagittal split setback
SSSS	staphylococcal scalded skin syndrome
SST	sagittal sinus thrombosis
SSX	sulfisoxazole acetyl
S/SX	signs/symptoms
ST	esotropic
	sacrum transverse
	shock therapy
	sinus tachycardia
	skin test
	slight trace
	speech therapist
	split thickness
	stomach
	straight
	stress testing
	stretcher
	subtotal
STA	second trimester abortion
	superficial temporal artery
stab.	polymorphonuclear leukocytes (white blood cells, in nonmature form)
STAI	State-Trait Anxiety Inventory
STAI-I	State-Trait-Anxiety Index—I
staph	*Staphylococcus aureus*
stat	immediately
STB	stillborn
STBAL	standing balance
ST BY	stand by
STC	serum theophylline concentration
	stimulate to cry
	subtotal colectomy
	sugar tongue cast
STD	sexually transmitted diseases
	skin test dose
	skin to tumor distance
	sodium tetradecylsulfate
STD TF	standard tube feeding
STEAM	stimulated-echo acquisition mode
STET	single photon emission tomography
	submaximal treadmill exercise test
STETH	stethoscope
STF	special tube feeding
	standard tube feeding
STG	short-term goals
	split-thickness graft

STH	soft tissue hemorrhage
	somatotrophic hormone
	subtotal hysterectomy
	supplemental thyroid hormone
STI	soft tissue injury
STJ	subtalar joint
STK	streptokinase
STL	serum theophylline level
STLE	St. Louis encephalitis
STLOM	swelling, tenderness, and limitation of motion
STM	short-term memory
	streptomycin
STNM	surgical-evaluative staging of cancer
STNR	symmetrical tonic neck reflex
STORCH	syphilis, toxoplasmosis, other agents, rubella, cytomegalovirus, and herpes (maternal infections)
STP	sodium thiopental
STPD	standard temperature and pressure-dry
STR	stretcher
strep	*streptococcus*
	streptomycin
STS	serologic test for syphilis
	sodium tetradecyl sulfate
	soft tissue swelling
STSG	split thickness skin graft
STT	scaphoid, trapezium trapezoid
	skin temperature test
STTOL	standing tolerance
STU	shock trauma unit
STV	short term variability
STZ	streptozocin
S&U	supine and upright
SU	sensory urgency
	Somogyi units
SUA	serum uric acid
	single umbilical artery
SUB	Skene's urethra and Bartholins glands
SUBL	sublingual
Subcu	subcutaneous
sub q	subcutaneous (this is a dangerous abbreviation since the q is mistaken for every, when a number follows)
SUD	sudden unexpected death
SUDS	Subjective Unit of Distress Scale
SUI	stress urinary incontinence
	suicide
SUID	sudden unexplained infant death
SULF-PRIM	trimethoprim and sulfamethoxazole
SUN	serum urea nitrogen
SUP	superior
	supination
	supinator
	symptomatic uterine prolapse
supp	suppository
SUR	surgery, surgical
Surgi	surgigator
SUUD	sudden unexpected, unexplained death
SUX	succinylcholine
	suction
SV	seminal vesical
	sigmoid volvulus
	single ventricle
	stock volume
SVB	saphenous vein bypass
SVC	slow vital capacity
	superior vena cava
SVCO	superior vena cava obstruction
SVCS	superior vena cava syndrome
SVD	single vessel disease
	spontaneous vaginal delivery
SVE	sterile vaginal examination
	Streptococcus viridans endocarditis
SVG	saphenous vein graft
SVL	severe visual loss
SVN	small volume nebulizer

SVO_2	mixed venous oxygen saturation
SVP	spontaneous venous pulse
SVPB	supraventricular premature beat
SVPC	supraventricular premature contraction
SVR	supraventricular rhythm
	systemic vascular resistance
SVRI	systemic vascular resistance index
SVT	supraventricular tachycardia
SW	sandwich
	Social Worker
	stab wound
SWD	short wave diathermy
SWFI	sterile water for injection
SWG	standard wire gauge
SWI	sterile water for injection
S&WI	surgical wound infection
	skin and wound isolation
SWOG	Southwest Oncology Group
SWP	small whirlpool
SWS	slow wave sleep
	student ward secretary
	Sturge-Weber syndrome
SWT	stab wound of the throat
SWU	septic work-up
Sx	signs
	surgery
	symptom
SXR	skull X-ray
syr	syrup
SYS BP	systolic blood pressure
SZ	schizophrenic
	seizure
	suction
SZN	streptozocin

T

T	tablespoon (15 mL) (this is a dangerous abbreviation)
	temperature
	tender
	tension
	testicles
	thoracic
	trace
t	teaspoon (5 mL) (this is a dangerous abbreviation)
T+	increase tension
$T_{1/2}$	half-life
T_1	tricuspid first sound
T_3	triiodithyronine
T-	decreased tension
T-2	dactinomycin, doxorubicin, vincristine, and cyclophosphamide
T3	Tylenol® with codeine 30 mg (this is a dangerous abbreviation)
T_4	levothyroxine
	thyroxine
$T_{3/4}$ind	triiodoithyronine to thyroxine index
T-7	free thyroxine factor
$T_1 \ldots T_{12}$	thoracic nerve 1 through 12
	thoracic vertebra 1 through 12
TA	Takayasu's arteritis
	temperature axillary
	temporal arteritis
	therapeutic abortion
	tracheal aspirate
	traffic accident
	tricuspid atresia
Ta	tonometry applanation
T&A	tonsillectomy and adenoidectomy
T(A)	axillary temperature
TAA	thoracic aortic aneurysm
	total ankle arthroplasty
	transverse aortic arch
	triamcinolone acetonide
	tumor associated antigen (antibodies)
TAB	tablet
	therapeutic abortion
	triple antibiotic (bacitracin, neomycin, and polymyxin—this is

a dangerous abbreviation)

TAC tetracaine, Adrenalin® and cocaine
triamicinolone cream

TAD transverse abdominal diameter

TADAC therapeutic abortion, dilation, aspiration, and curettage

TAE transcatheter arterial embolization

TAF tissue angiogenesis factor

TAH total abdominal hysterectomy
total artificial heart

TAHBSO total abdominal hysterectomy, bilateral salpingo-oophorectomy

TAL tendon Achilles lengthening
total arm length

TAML therapy-related acute myelogenous leukemia

TAM tamoxifen
teenage mother

TANI total axial (lymph) node irradiation

TAO thromboangitis obliterans
troleandomycin

TAP tonometry by applanation

TAPVC total anomalous pulmonary venous connection

TAPVD total anomalous pulmonary venous drainage

TAPVR total anomalous pulmonary venous return

TAR thrombocytopenia with absent radius
total ankle replacement
treatment authorization request

TARA total articular replacement arthroplasty

TAS therapeutic activities specialist
typical absence seizures

TAT tetanus antitoxin
till all taken
Thematic Apperception Test

TB total base
total bilirubin
total body
tuberculosis

TBA to be absorbed
to be added
to be admitted
total body (surface) area

TBB transbronchial biopsy

tbc tuberculosis

TBE tick-born encephalitis

TBF total body fat

TBG thyroxine-binding globulin

TBI toothbrushing instruction
total body irradiation

T bili total bilirubin

TBK total body potassium

tbl. tablespoon (15 mL)

TBLB transbronchial lung biopsy

TBLC term birth, living child

TBLF term birth, living female

TBLM term birth, living male

TBM tracheobronchomalacia
tubule basement membrane

TBNA total body sodium
transbronchial needle aspiration
treated but not admitted

TBP total-body photographs

TBPA thyroxine-binding prealbumin

TBR total bed rest

TBSA total burn surface area

tbsp tablespoon (15 mL)

TBT tolbutamide test
tracheal bronchial toilet

TBV total blood volume
transluminal balloon valvuloplasty

TBW total body water

TBX_2 thromboxane B2

TBX® thiabendazole

TC throat culture
tissue culture

	transcobalamin
	trauma center
	true conjugate
	tubocurarine
Tc	technetium
T/C	telephone call
	to consider
T&C	turn and cough
	type and crossmatch
T&C#3	Tylenol® with 30 mg codeine
TCA	team conference
	terminal cancer
	thioguianine and cytarabine
	trichloroacetic acid
	tricuspid atresia
	tricyclic antidepressant
TCABG	triple coronary artery bypass graft
TCAD	tricyclic antidepressant
TCBS agar	thiosulfate-citrate-bile salt-sucrose agar
TCC	transitional cell carcinoma
TCD	transverse cardiac diameter
TCCB	transitional cell carcinoma of bladder
TCDB	turn, cough, and deep breath
TCDD	tetrachlorodibenzo-p-dioxin
TCE	tetrachloroethylene
T cell	small lymphocyte
TCH	turn, cough, hyperventilate
TCID	tissue culture infective dose
TCM	tissue culture media
	traditional Chinese medicine
	transcutaneous monitor
TCMH	tumor-direct cell-mediated hypersensitivity
TCMZ	trichloromethiazide
TCN	tetracycline
TCNS	transcutaneous nerve stimulator
TCNU	tauromustine
TcO_4	pertechnetate
TCOM	transcutaneous oxygen monitor
$TcPCO_2$	transcutaneous carbon dioxide
$TcPO_2$	transcutaneous oxygen
TCT	thyrocalcitonin
TCVA	thromboembolic cerebral vascular accident
TD	Takayasu's disease
	tardive dyskinesia
	tetanus-diphtheria toxoid (pediatric use)
	tidal volume
	tone decay
	transverse diameter
	travelers diarrhea
	treatment discontinued
Td	tetanus-diphtheria toxoid (adult type)
TDD	thoracic duct drainage
TDE	total daily energy (requirement)
TDF	tumor dose fractionation
TDI	toluene diisocyanate
TDK	tardive diskinesia
TDL	thoracic duct lymph
TDM	therapeutic drug monitoring
TDN	transdermal nitroglycerin
TDNTG	transdermal nitroglycerin
TdP	torsade de pointes
TdR	Thymidine
TDT	tentative discharge tomorrow
TDWB	touch down weight bearing
TDx®	fluorescence polarization immunoassay
TE	echo time
	tennis elbow
	trace elements
	tracheoesophageal
T&E	trial and error
TEA	thromboendarterectomy
	total elbow arthroplasty
TEC	total eosinophil count
T&EC	trauma and emergency center
TEDS®	Anti-embolism Stockings

TEE	transesophageal echocardiography
TEF	tracheoesophageal fistula
TEG	thromboelastogram
TEI	transesophageal imaging
TEL	telemetry
tele	telemetry
TEM	transmission electron microscopy
TEN	tension (intraocular pressure)
	toxic epidermal necrolysis
TEN®	Total Enteral Nutrition
TENS	transcutaneous electrical nerve stimulation
TEP	tracheoesophageal puncture
	tubal ectopic pregnancy
TER	total elbow replacement
TERB	terbutaline
tert.	tertiary
TES	Treatment Emergent Symptoms
TESPA	thiotepa
TET	transcranial electrostimulation therapy
	treadmill exercise test
TF	tactile fremitus
	tetralogy of Fallot
	to follow
	tube feeding
TFB	trifascicular block
TFL	tensor fascia lata
TFT	trifluridine (trifluorothymidine)
TFTs	thyroid function tests
TG	triglycerides
6-TG	thioguanine
TGA	transient global amnesia
	transposition of the great arteries
TGFA	triglyceride fatty acid
TGS	tincture of green soap
TGT	thromboplastin generation test
TGV	thoracic gas volume
TGXT	thallium-graded exercise test
TH	thrill
	thyroid hormone
	total hysterectomy
T&H	type and hold
THA	tacrine (tetrahydroacridine)
	total hip arthroplasty
	transient hemispheric attack
THAM®	tromethamine
THC	tetrahydrocannibinol (dronabinol)
	transhepatic cholangiogram
TH-CULT	throat culture
THE	transhepatic embolization
Ther Ex	therapeutic exercise
THI	transient hypogammaglobinemia of infancy
THKAFO	trunk-hip-knee-ankle-foot orthosis
THP	take home packs
	trihexphenidyl
THR	total hip replacement
	training heart rate
TI	tricuspid insufficiency
TIA	transient ischemic attack
tib.	tibia
TIBC	total iron-binding capacity
TIC	trypsin-inhibitor capacity
TID	three times a day
TIE	transient ischemic episode
TIG	tetanus immune globulin
TIL	tumor-infiltrating lymphocytes
TIN	three times a night (this is a dangerous abbreviation)
tinct	tincture
TIS	tumor *in situ*
TISS	Therapeutic Intervention Scoring System
TIT	Treponema (pallidum) immobilization test
	triiodothyronine
TIVC	thoracic inferior vena cava
+tive	positive
TIW	three times a week (this is a dangerous abbreviation)
TJ	triceps jerk

TJA	total joint arthroplasty
TJN	twin jet nebulizer
TK	thymidine kinase
TKA	total knee arthroplasty
TKD	tokodynamometer
TKE	terminal knee extension
TKNO	to keep needle open
TKP	thermokeratoplasty
TKO	to keep open
TKR	total knee replacement
TKVO	to keep vein open
TL	team leader trial leave tubal ligation
Tl	thallium
TLA	translumbar arteriogram (aortogram)
T/L	terminal latency
TLC	tender loving care thin layer chromatography total lung capacity total lymphocyte count triple lumen catheter
TLD	thermoluminescent dosimeter
TLI	total lymphoid irradiation translaryngeal intubation
TLNB	term living newborn
TLP	transitional living program
TLR	tonic labyrinthine reflex
TLS	tumor lysis syndrome
TLSO	thoracic lumbar sacral orthosis
TLSSO	thoracolumbosacral spinal orthosis
TLV	total lung volume
TM	temperature by mouth Thayer Martin (culture) trabecular meshwork transcendental meditation tumor tympanic membrane
T & M	type and crossmatch
TMA	thrombotic microangiopathy transmetatarsal amputation
TMB	transient monocular blindness trimethoxybenzoates
TMC	transmural colitis triamicinolone
TME	thermolysin-like metalleondopeptidase
TMET	tread mill exercise test
TMI	threatened myocardial infarction
TMJ	temporomandibular joint
TMM	torn medial meniscus
Tmm	McKay-Marg tension
TMP	thallium myocardial perfusion transmembrane pressure trimethoprim
TMP/SMX	trimethoprimsulfamethoxazole
TMR	trainable mentally retarded
TMST	treadmill stress test
TMT	treadmill test
TMTC	too many to count
TMTX	trimethexate
TMX	tamoxifen
TMZ	temazepam
TN	normal intraocular tension team nursing temperature normal
T&N	tension and nervousness
TNA	total nutrient admixture
TNB	term newborn Tru-Cut® needle biopsy
TNF	tumor necrosis factor
TNG	nitroglycerin
TNI	total nodal irradiation
TNM	primary tumor, regional lymph nodes, and distant metastasis (used with subscripts for the staging of cancer)
TNS	transcutaneous nerve stimulation (stimulator)
TNT	tramcinolone and nystatin
TNTC	too numerous to count
TO	old tuberculin telephone order total obstruction transfer out
T(O)	oral temperature
T&O	tubes and ovaries

TOA	time of arrival
	tubo-ovarian abscess
TOB	tobramycin
TOCE	transcatheter oily chemoembolization
TOCO	tocodynamometer
TOD	intraocular pressure of the right eye
TOF	tetralogy of Fallot
	total of four
TOGV	transposition of the great vessels
TOH	throughout hospitalization
TOL	trial of labor
TOM	tomorrow
	transcutaneous oxygen monitor
Tomo	tomography
TON	tonight
TOP	termination of pregnancy
TOPV	trivalent oral polio vaccine
TORCH	toxoplasmosis, other (syphillis, hepatitis, Zoster), rubella,cy-tomegalovirus, and herpes simplex (maternal infections)
TORP	total ossicular replacement prosthesis
TOS	intraocular pressure of the left eye
	thoracic outlet syndrome
TOT BILI	total bilirubin
TP	temperature and pressure
	temporoparietal
	therapeutic pass
	thrombophlebitis
	Todd's paralysis
	total protein
	treating physician
T & P	temperature and pulse
	turn and position
TPA	alteplase, recombinant (tissue plasminogen activator)
	tissue polypeptide antigen
	total parenteral alimentation
TPC	total patient care
TPD	tropical pancreatic diabetes
TPE	therapeutic plasma exchange
	total protective environment
TPF	trained participating father
TPH	thromboembolic pulmonary hypertension
	trained participating husband
T PHOS	triple phosphate crystals
TPI	*Treponema pallidium* immobilization
T plasty	tympanoplasty
TPM	temporary pacemaker
TPN	total parenteral nutrition
TP & P	time, place, and person
TPO	thrombopoietin
	trial prescription order
TPPN	total peripheral parenteral nutrition
	trans pars plana vitrectomy
TPR	temperature
	temperature, pulse, and respiration
	total peripheral resistance
T PROT	total protein
TPT	time to peak tension
	treadmill performance test
TPVR	total peripheral vascular resistance
TR	therapeutic recreation
	tincture
	to return
	trace
	transfusion reaction
	transplant recipients
	treatment
	tricuspid regurgitation
	tremor
	tumor registry
T(R)	rectal temperature
T & R	tenderness and rebound
TRA	therapeutic recreation associate
	to run at

trach. tracheal
tracheostomy
Trans D transverse diameter
TRAS transplant renal artery stenosis
TRC tanned red cells
TRD tongue-retaining device
traction retinal detachment
Tren Trendelenberg
TRH protirelin (thyrotropin-releasing hormone)
TRI trimester
TRIG triglycerides
TRISS Trauma Score and Injury Severity Score
TRM-SMX trimethoprimsulfamethoxazole
tRNA transfer ribonucleic acid
TRND Trendelenburg
TRO to return to office
TRP tubular reabsorption of phosphate
TRS Therapeutic Recreation Specialist
TRT thermoradiotherapy
T3RU triiodothyroxine resin uptake
TRUS transrectal ultrasound
TRUSP transrectal ultrasound of the prostate
TRZ triazolam
TS temperature sensitive
test solution
toe signs
Tourette's syndrome
transsexual
Trauma Score
tricuspid stenosis
TSA toluenesulfonic acid
total shoulder arthroplasty
TSAR® tape surrounded Appli-rulers
TSBB transtracheal selective bronchial brushing
TSC technetium sulfur colloid
theophylline serum concentration
TSD target to skin distance
Tay-Sachs disease
T set tracheotomy set
TSE testicular self-examination
TSF tricep skin fold
TSH thyroid-stimulating hormone
tsp teaspoon (5 mL)
TSP total serum protein
TSPA thiotepa
TSR total shoulder replacement
TSS toxic shock syndrome
TST titmus stereocuity test
trans-scrotal testosterone
treadmill stress test
T&T tobramycin and ticarcillin
touch and tone
TT tetanus toxoid
thrombin time
thymol turbidity
tilt table
tonometry
transtracheal
twitch tension
T/T trace of ___ /trace of___
TT4 total thyroxine
TTA total toe arthroplasty
TTD temporary total disability
transverse thoracic diameter
TTN transient tachypnea of the newborn
TTNA transthoracic needle aspiration
TTNB transient tachypnea of the newborn
TTO to take out
transtracheal oxygen
TTOD tetanus toxoid outdated
TTOT transtracheal oxygen therapy
TTP thrombotic thrombocytopenic purpura
TTR triceps tendon reflex
TTS tarsal tunnel syndrome
temporary threshold shift
through the skin
transdermal therapeutic system
TTT tolbutamide tolerance test

TTUTD tetanus toxoid up-to-date
TTVP temporary transvenous pacemaker
TTWB touch toe weight bearing
TU Todd units
transrectal ultrasound
tuberculin units
TUF total ultrafiltration
TUN total urinary nitrogen
TUPR transurethral prostatic resection
TUR transurethral resection
T_3UR triiodothyronine uptake ratio
TURB turbidity
TURBN transurethral resection bladder neck
TURBT transurethral resection bladder tumor
TURP transurethral resection of prostate
TURV transurethral resection valves
TUU transureteroureterostomy
TV television
temporary visit
tidal volume
transvenous
trial visit
Trichomonas vaginalis
T/V touch-verbal
TVC triple voiding cystogram
true vocal cord
TVDALV triple vessel disease with an abnormal left ventricle
TVF tactile vocal fremitus
TVH total vaginal hysterectomy
TVN tonic vibration response
TVP transvenous pacemaker
transvesicle prostatectomy
TVSC transvaginal sector scan
TVU total volume of urine
TVUS transvaginal ultrasound
TW tapwater
test weight
TWD total white and differential count
TWE tapwater enema
TWETC tapwater enema till clear
TWG total weight gain
TWHW ok toe walking and heel walking all right
TWR total wrist replacement
TWWD tap water wet dressing
Tx therapy
traction
transfuse
transplant
treatment
tympanostomy
T & X type and crossmatch
TxA_2 thromboxane A_2
TXM type and crossmatch
T cell crossmatch
TYCO #3 Tylenol® with 30 mg of codeine (#1=7.5 mg, #2=15 mg and#4=60 mg of codeine present
Tyl Tylenol®
tyloma (callus)
TYMP tympanogram
TZ transition zone

U

U ultralente insulin
units (this is the most dangerous abbreviation —spell out "unit")
urine
U/1 1 finger breadth below umbilicus
1/U 1 finger over umbilicus
U/ at umbilicus
UA umbilical artery
unauthorized absence
uncertain about
upper arm
upper airway
uric acid
urinalysis
UAC umbilical artery catheter
under active
upper airway congestion
UAL umbilical artery line
up *ad lib*
UAO upper airway obstruction
UAPF upon arrival patient found
UAT up as tolerated

UAVC	univentricular atrioventricular connection
UBF	unknown black female
UBI	ultraviolet blood irradiation
UBM	unknown black male
UBW	usual body weight
UC	ulcerative colitis
	umbilical cord
	unconscious
	urea clearance
	urine culture
	uterine contraction
U&C	urethral & cervical
	usual and customary
UCD	urine collection device
	usual childhood diseases
UCE	urea cycle enzymopathy
UCG	urinary chorionicgonado-tropins
UCHD	usual childhood diseases
UCHS	uncontrolled hemorrhagic shock
UCI	urethral catheter in
	usual childhood illnesses
UCL	uncomfortable loudness level
UCO	urethral catheter out
UCP	urethral closure pressure
UCR	unconditioned response
	usual, customary, and reasonable
UCRE	urine creatinine
UCS	unconscious
UCX	urine culture
UD	as directed
	urethral discharge
	uterine distension
UDC	usual diseases of childhood
UDCA	ursodeoxycholic acid
UDN	updraft nebulizer
UDO	undetermined origin
UDS	unconditioned stimulus
UE	under elbow
	undetermined etiology
	upper extremity
UES	upper esophageal sphincter
UESP	upper esophageal sphincter pressure
UF	ultrafiltration
	until finished
UFC	urine-free cortisol
UFF	unusual facial features
UFFI	urea formaldehyde foam insulation
UFN	until further notice
UFO	unflagged order
UFR	ultrafiltration rate
UG	until gone
	urinary glucose
	urogenital
UGDP	University Group Diabetes Project
UGH	uveitis, glaucoma, and hyphema
UGI	upper gastrointestinal series
UGIH	upper gastrointestinal (tract) hemorrhage
UGK	urine glucose ketones
UH	umbilical hernia
	University Hospital
UHBI	upper hemibody irradiation
UHDDS	Uniform Hospital Discharge Data Set
UHP	University Health Plan
UI	urinary incontinence
UIBC	unsaturated iron binding capacity
UID	once daily (this is a dangerous abbreviation, spell out "once daily")
UIQ	upper inner quadrant
UK	unknown
	urine potassium
	urokinase
U/L	upper and lower
U & L	upper and lower
ULLE	upper lid, left eye
ULN	upper limits of normal
ULQ	upper left quadrant
ULRE	upper lid, right eye
ULYTES	electrolytes, urine
UM	unmarried
umb ven	umbilical vein
UN	undernourished

	urinary nitrogen
UNA	urinary nitrogen appearance
UNa	urine sodium
unacc	unaccompanied
ung	ointment
UNK	unknown
UNOS	United Network of Organ Sharing
UO	under observation
	undetermined origin
	urinary output
UOP	urinary output
UOQ	upper outer quadrant
Uosm	urinary osmolality
✓ up	check up
UP	unipolar
UPJ	ureteropelvic junction
UPOR	usual place of residence
UPPP	uvulopalatopharyngoplasty
U/P ratio	urine to plasma ratio
UPT	uptake
	urine pregnancy test
UR	utilization review
URD	undifferentiated respiratory disease
URI	upper respiratory infection
URIC A	uric acid
url	unrelated
UROB	urobilinogen
urol	urology
URQ	upper right quadrant
URTI	upper respiratory tract infection
US	ultrasonography
	unit secretary
USA	unit services assistant
	United States Army
USAF	United States Air Force
USAN	United States Adopted Names
USAP	unstable angina pectoris
USB	upper sternal border
USCVD	unsterile controlled vaginal delivery
USDA	United States Department of Agriculture
USG	ultrasonography
USH	usual state of health
USI	urinary stress incontinence
USMC	United States Marine Corp
USN	ultrasonic nebulizer
	United States Navy
USP	United States Pharmacopeia
USPHS	United States Public Health Service
USUCVD	unsterile uncontrolled vaginal delivery
USVMD	urine specimen volume measuring device
UTD	up to date
ut dict	as directed
UTF	usual throat flora
UTI	urinary tract infection
UTO	unable to obtain
	upper tibial osteotomy
UTS	ulnar tunnel syndrome
	ultrasound
UUN	urinary urea nitrogen
UV	ultraviolet
	ureterovesical
	urine volume
UVA	ultraviolet A light
	ureterovesical angle
UVB	ultraviolet B light
UVC	umbilical vein catheter
UVJ	ureterovesical junction
UVL	ultraviolet light
	umbilical venous line
UVR	ultraviolet radiation
U/WB	unit of whole blood
UW	unilateral weakness
UWF	unknown white female
UWM	unknown white male
	unwed mother

V

V	five
	gas volume
	minute volume
	vagina
	vein
	verb
	vomiting
$\dot{v}$	Ventilation (L/min)

+V	positive vertical divergence
V&C	vertical and centric (a bite)
V_1 to V_6	precordial chest leads
VA	vacuum aspiration
	valproic acid
	Veterans Administration
	visual acuity
V_A	minute alveolar ventilation
VAB	vinblastine, dactinomycin, bleomycin, cisplatin, and cyclophosphamide
VAC	ventriculo-arterial connections
	vincristine, dactinomycin, and cyclophosphamide
	vincristine, doxorubicin, and cyclophosphamide
VAD	vascular (venous) access device
	vincristine, doxorubicin, and dexamethasone
VADRIAC	vincristine, doxorubicin, and cyclophosphamide
vag.	vagina
VAG HYST	vaginal hysterectomy
VAH	Veterans Administration Hospital
VAIN	vaginal intrapiethelial neoplasia
VALE	visual acuity, left eye
VAMC	Veterans Administration Medical Center
VAMS	Visual Analogue Mood Scale
VANCO/P	vancomycin-peak
VANCO/T	vancomycin trough
VAP	venous access port
	vincristine, asparaginase, and prednisone
VAR	variant
VARE	visual acuity, right eye
VAS	vascular
	visual analogue scale
VASC	Visual-Auditory Screen Test for Children
VAS RAD	vascular radiology
VATER	vertebral, anal, tracheal, esophageal and renal anomalies
VATH	vinblastine, doxorubicin, thiotepa, and fluoxymesterone
VB	Van Buren (catheter)
	venous blood
	vinblastine and methotrexate
VB_1	first voided bladder specimen
VB_2	second midstream bladder specimen
VBAC	vaginal birth after cesarean
VBAP	vincristine, carmustine, doxorubicin, and prednisone
VBC	vinblastine, bleomycin, and cisplatin
VBD	vinblastine, bleomycin, and cisplatin
VBG	venous blood gas
	vertical banded gastroplasty
VBI	vertebrobasilar insufficiency
VBL	vinblastine
VBP	vinblastine, bleomycin, and cisplatin
VBS	vertebral-basilar system
VC	color vision
	etoposide and carboplatin
	pulmonary capillary blood volume
	vena cava
	vital capacity
	vocal cords
VCAP	vincristine, cyclophosphamide, doxorubicin, and prednisone
VCCA	velocity common carotid artery
VCG	vectocardiography
VCO	centilator CPAP oxyhood
VCR	vincristine sulfate
VCT	venous clotting time
VCU	voiding cystourethrogram

VCUG	vesicoureterogram
	voiding cystourethrogram
VD	venereal disease
	voided
	volume of distribution
V_D	deadspace volume
V&D	vomiting and diarrhea
VDA	venous digital angiogram
	visual discriminatory acuity
VDAC	vaginal delivery after cesarean
VDD	atrial synchronous ventricular inhibited pacing
VDG	venereal disease—gonorrhea
Vdg	voiding
VDH	valvular disease of the heart
VDL	vasodepressor lipid
	visual detection level
VD or M	venous distention or masses
VDP	vinblastine, decarbazine, and cisplatin
VDRL	Venereal Disease Research Laboratory (test for syphilis)
VDRR	vitamin D-resistant rickets
VDS	venereal disease—syphilis
	vindesine
VDT	video display terminal
VD/VT	dead space to tidal volume ratio
VE	vaginal examination
	vertex
	vocational evaluation
V_E	minute volume (expired)
VEA	ventricular ectopic activity
VEB	ventricular ectopic beat
VED	ventricular ectopic depolarization
VEE	Venezuelan equine encephalitis
VENT	ventilation
	ventilator
	ventral
	ventricular
VEP	visual evoked potential
VER	ventricular escape rhythm
	visual evoked responses
VET	veteran
VF	left leg (electrode)
	ventricular fibrillation
	vision field
	vocal fremitus
VFI	visual fields intact
V. Fib	ventricular fibrillation
VFP	vitreous fluorophotometry
VFPN	Volu-feed premie nipple
VFRN	Volu-feed regular nipple
VG	vein graft
	ventricular gallop
	very good
VGH	very good health
VH	vaginal hysterectomy
	Veterans Hospital
	viral hepatitis
	vitreous hemorrhage
VHD	valvular heart disease
VI	six
	volume index
vib	vibration
VICA	velocity internal carotid artery
VID	videodensitometry
VIG	vaccinia immune globulin
VIN	vaginal intra-epiheal neoplasia
VIP	etopside, ifosfamide, and cisplatin
	vasoactive intestinal peptide
	vasoactive intracorpeal pharmacotherapy
	very important patient
	vinblastine, ifosfamide, and cisplatin
	voluntary interruption of pregnancy
VISC	vitreous infusion suction cutter
VIT	venom immunotherapy
	vital
	vitamin
vit. cap.	vital capacity
VIZ	namely
VKC	vernal keratoconjunctivitis

VL left arm (electrode)
VLBW very low birth weight
VLCD very low calorie diet
VLCFA very long chain fatty acids
VLDL very low density lipoprotein
VLH ventrolateral nucleus of the hypothalamus
VM 26 teniposide
VMA vanillylmandelic acid
VMCP vincristine, melphalan, cyclophosphamide, and prednisone
VMH ventromedial hypothalamus
VMO vastic medalis oblique
VMR vasomotor rhinitis
VN visiting nurse
VNA Visiting Nurses' Association
VNC vesicle neck contracture
VO verbal order
VOCAB vocabulary
VOCTOR void on call to operating room
VOD venocclusive disease
vision right eye
VOL volume
voluntary
VOO continuous ventricular asynchronous pacing
VOR vestibular ocular reflex
VOS vision left eye
VOT Visual Organization Test
VOU vision both eyes
VP etoposide
variegate porphyria
venous pressure
ventricularoperitoneal
ventricul-peritoneal
V & P vagotomy and pyloroplasty
ventilation and perfusion
VP-16 etoposide
VPA valproic acid
VPB ventricular premature beat
VPC ventricular premature contractions
VPDF vegetable protein diet plus fiber
VPDs ventricular premature depolarizations
VPI velopharyngeal insufficiency
VPL vento-posterolateral
VPR volume pressure response
VQ ventilation perfusion
VR valve replacement
right arm (electrode)
ventricular rhythm
verbal reprimand
vocational rehabilitation
VRA visual reinforcement audiometry
VRC vocational rehabilitation counselor
VRI viral respiratory infection
VRL ventral root, lumbar
VRT variance of resident time
ventral root, thoracic
Visual Retention Test
VS versus
very sensitive
vital signs
VSBE very short below elbow (cast)
VSD ventricular septal defect
VSI visual motor integration
VSO vertical subcondylar oblique
VSOK vital signs normal
VSR venous stasis retinopathy
VSS vital signs stable
VT ventricular tachycardia
v. tach. ventricular tachycardia
VTE venous thromboembolism
VTEC verotoxin-producing *Escherichia coli*
VTX vertex
VV varicose veins
V&V vulva and vagina
V/V volume to volume ratio
VVD vaginal vertex delivery
VVFR vesicovaginal fistula repair
V/VI grade 5 on a 6 grade basis

VVOR visual-vestibulo-ocular-reflex
VVT ventricular synchronous pacing
VW vessel wall
VWD von Willebrand's disease
VWM ventricular wall motion
V_x vitrectomy
VZ varicella zoster
VZIG varicella zoster immune globulin
VZV varicella zoster virus

W

w week
weight
white
widowed
wife
with
WA when awake
while awake
wide awake
W or A weakness or atrophy
WAF weakness, atrophy, and fasciculation
white adult female
WAIS Wechsler Adult Intelligence Scale
WAIS-R Wechsler Adult Intelligence Scale-Revised
WAM white adult male
WAP wandering atrial pacemaker
WAS Wishott-Aldrich syndrome
WASS Wasserman test
WAT word association test
WB waist belt
weight bearing
well baby
Western blot
whole blood
WBAT weight bearing as tolerated
WBC well baby clinic
white blood cell (count)
WBCT whole blood clotting time
WBH whole-body hyperthermia
W Bld whole blood
WBN wellborn nursery
WBQC wide base quad cane
WBR whole body radiation
WBS whole body scan
WBTF Waring Blender tube feeding
WBTT weight bearing to tolerance
WBUS weeks by ultrasound
WC ward clerk
ward confinement
wet compresses
wheelchair
white count
whooping cough
will call
WCC well child care
white cell count
WD ward
well developed
well differentiated
wet dressing
Wilson's disease
word
wound
W/D warm and dry
withdrawal
W→D wet to dry
W4D Worth four-dot (test)
WDCC well-developed collateral circulation
WDF white divorced female
WDHA watery diarrhea, hypokalemia, and achlorhydria
WDLL well-differentiated lymphocytic lymphoma
WDM white divorced male
WDWN-BM well-developed, well-nourished black male
WDWN-WF well-developed, well-nourished white female
WE weekend
W/E weekend
WEE Western equine encephalitis
WEP weekend pass

WF	white female
WFI	water for injection
WFL	within functional limits
WF-O	will follow in office
WFR	wheel-and-flare reaction
WH	walking heel (cast)
WHO	World Health Organization
	wrist-hand orthosis
WHPB	whirlpool bath
WHV	woodchuck hepatitis virus
WHVP	wedged hepatic venous pressure
WI	ventricular demand pacing
	walk-in
W/I	within
W+I	work and interest
WIA	wounded in action
WIC	women, infants, and children
WID	widow
	widower
WISC	Wechsler Intelligence Scale for Children
WISC-R	Weschler Intelligence Scale for Children-revised
wk	week
WL	waiting list
	weight loss
WLS	wet lung syndrome
WLT	waterload test
WK	week
	work
WKS	Wernicke-Korsakoff syndrome
WM	white male
WMA	wall motion abnormality
WMF	white married female
WMM	white married male
WMP	weight management program
WMX	whirlpool, massage, and exercise
WN	well nourished
WND	wound
WNL	within normal limits
WNLS	weighted nonlinear least squares
WO	weeks old
	written order
W/O	water in oil
	without
WOP	without pain
W.P.	whirlpool
WPFM	Wright peak flow meter
WPP	Welcher Preschool Primary Scale of Intelligence
WPPSI	Wechsler Preschool and Primary Scale of Intelligence
WPW	Wolff-Parkinson-White
WR	Wasserman reaction
	wrist
WRAT	Wide Range Achievement Test
WS	ward secretary
	watt seconds
	work simplification
W&S	wound and skin
WSepF	white separated female
WSepM	white separated male
WSF	white single female
WSM	white single male
WSP	wearable speech processor
WT	walking tank
	weight (wt)
	wisdom teeth
WTS	whole tomography slice
W/U	workup
WV	whispered voice
W/V	weight-to-volume ratio
WW	Weight Watchers
W/W	weight-to-weight ratio
WWAC	walk with aid of cane
WWidF	white widowed female
WWidM	white widowed male

X

X	break
	cross
	crossmatch
	except
	start of anesthesia
	ten
	times
	xylocaine
X̄	except

X^2	chi-square
X+#	xyphoid plus number of fingerbreadths
X3	orientation as to time, place and person
XBT	xylose breath test
XC	excretory cystogram
XD	times daily
X&D	examination and diagnosis
X2d	times two days
XDP	xeroderma pigmentosum
Xe	xenon
XeCT	xenon-enhance computed tomography
X-ed	crossed
XKO	not knocked out
XL	extra large
X-leg	cross leg
XLH	X-linked hypophos-phatemia
XLJR	X-linked juvenile retinoschisis
XM	crossmatch
X-mat.	crossmatch
XMM	xeromammography
XOM	extraocular movements
XP	xeroderma pigmentosum
XR	x-ray
XRT	radiation therapy
XS	excessive
XS-LIM	exceeds limits of procedure
XT	exotropia
X(T)	intermittent exotropia
XU	excretory urogram
XULN	times upper limit of normal
XV	fifteen
XX	normal female sex chromosome type twenty
XX/XY	sex karyotypes
XXX	thirty
XY	normal male sex chromosome type
XYL	Xylocaine
XYLO	xylocaine

Y

YACP	young adult chronic patient
YAG	yittrium aluminum garnert (laser)
Yb	ytterbium
Yel	yellow
YF	yellow fever
YFI	yellow fever immunization
YJV	yellow jacket venom
YLC	youngest living child
Y/N	yes/no
YO	years old
YOB	year of birth
YORA	younger-onset rheumatoid arthritis
YPLL	years of potential life lost before age 65
yr	year
YSC	yolk sac carcinoma
YTD	year to date

Z

Z-E	Zollinger-Ellison (syndrome)
ZEEP	zero end-expiratory pressure
ZES	Zellinger-Ellison syndrome
Z-ESR	zeta erythrocyte sedimentation rate
ZIG	zoster serum immune globulin
ZIP	zoster immune plasma
ZMC	zygomatic
Zn	zinc
ZnO	zinc oxide
ZnOE	zinc oxide & eugenol
ZPC	zero point of charge zopiclone
ZPO	zinc peroxide
ZPT	zinc pyrithione
ZSB	zero stools since birth
ZSR	zeta sedimentation rate

Miscellaneous

↑	above
	alive
	elevated
	greater than
	high
	improved
	increase
	rising
↓	dead
	decrease
	falling
	lowered
	normal plantar reflex
	restricted
→	causes to
	progressing
	results in
	showed
	to the right
←	resulted from
	to the left
⟷	stable
	to and from
	unchanging
↓↓	flexor
	testes descended
↑↑	extensor
	positive Babinsky
	testes undescended
‖	parallel
	parallel bars
✓	check
	flexion
#	fracture
	number
	pound
∴	therefore
Δ scan	delta scan (computed tomography scan)
+	plus
	positive
	present
—	absent
	minus
	negative
/	slash mark signifying per, and, or with

	(this is a dangerous symbol as it is mistaken for a one)
±	either positive or negative
	no definite cause
	plus or minus
	very slight trace
	right lower quadrant
┌	right upper quadrant
┐	left upper quadrant
┘	left lower quadrant
>	greater than
≥	greater than or equal to
<	caused by
	less than
≤	less than or equal to
≮	not less than
≯	not more than
∧	above
	diastolic blood pressure
	increased
∨	below
	systolic blood pressure
≠	not equal to
≅	approximately equal to
≈	approximately
×	left ear-air conduction threshold
>	left ear-bone conduction threshold
□	left ear-masked air conduction threshold
]	left ear-masked bone conduction threshold
○	right ear-air conduction threshold
<	right ear-bone conduction threshold
△	right ear-masked air conduction threshold
[	right ear-masked bone conduction

⊖	threshold
	threshold
	reversible
?	questionable
∅	no
	none
@	at
1°	first degree
	primary
2°	second degree
	secondary
3°	tertiary
	third degree
i	one (Roman numerals are dangerous expressions and should not be used)
ii	two
iii	three
iiii	four
iv	four (this is a dangerous abbreviation as it is read as intravenous, use 4)
v	five
vi	six
vii	seven
viii	eight
ix	nine
x	ten
xi	eleven
xii	twelve
♂	male
♀	female
■	deceased male
●	deceased female
□	living male
○	living female
◇	sex unknown
(□)	adopted living male
*	birth
†	dead
	death
⚲	standing
o—<	recumbent position

⚲ (bent)	sitting position
♥	heart
Α α	alpha
Β β	beta
Γ γ	gamma
Δ δ	anion gap
	change
	delta
	delta gap
	prism diopter
	temperature
	trimester
Ε ϵ	epsilon
Ζ ζ	zeta
Η η	eta
Θ θ	negative
	theta
Ι ι	iota
Κ κ	kappa
Λ λ	lambda
Μ μ	micro
	mu
Ν ν	nu
Ξ ξ	xi
Ο ο	omicron
Ππ	pi
Ρ ρ	rho
Σ σ	sigma
	sum of
Τ τ	tau
Υ υ	upsilon
Φ ϕ	phenyl
	phi
	thyroid
Χ χ	chi
Ψ ψ	psi
	psychiatric
Ω ω	omega
′	feet
	minutes (as in 30′)
″	inches
	seconds
⊙	start of an operation
⊗	end of anesthesia
3×	three times
2×2	gauze dressing folded 2″ x 2″
4×4	gauze dressing folded 4″ x 4″

140 | 101 | 17 Na = 140, Cl = 101, BUN = 17
3.4 | 25 | 140 K = 3.4, CO_2 = 25, glucose = 140

5.0 > 16 | 85 / 45 | 30 < 35 red blood cell count, hemoglobin, mean corpuscular volume, mean corpuscular hemoglobin concentration, hematocrit, mean corpuscular hemoglobin

2 cm | 80% / −2 Vtx

2 cm = dilation of cervix
80% = degree of cervix effacement
Vtx = vertex; presentation of fetus,
(breech = Br)
−2=station; distance above (−) or below (+) the spine of the ischium measured in cm

sodium | chloride | BUN < glucose
potassium | bicarbonate | creatinine.

calcium | protein | AST | LDH < bilirubin
phosphorus | albumin | ALT | Alkaline phos

segmented neutrophils | lymphocytes | eosinophils
banded neutrophils | monocytes | basophils

hemoglobin | WBC
hematocrit | platlets

Note: there are many individual variations as to how these are arranged

Reflexes[6]

Reflexes are usually graded on a 0 to 4+ scale:

4+ may indicate disease
often associated with clonus
very brisk, hyperactive
3+ brisker than average
possibly but not necessarily indicative of disease
2+ average
normal
1+ low normal
somewhat diminished
0 may indicate neuropathy
no response

Muscle strength[6]

0—No muscular contraction detected
1—A barely detectable flicker or trace of contraction
2—Active movement of the body part with gravity eliminated
3—Active movement against gravity
4—Active movement against gravity and some resistance
5—Active movement against full resistance without evident fatigue. This is normal muscle strength

Pulse[6]

0	completely absent
+1	markedly impaired
+2	moderately impaired
+3	slightly impaired
+4	normal

Gradation of intensity of heart murmurs[6]

1/6 or I/VI	may not be heard in all positions very faint, heard only after the listener has "tuned in"
2/6 or II/VI	quiet, but heard immediately upon placing the stethoscope on the chest
3/6 or III/VI	moderately loud
4/6 or IV/VI	loud
5/6 or V/VI	very loud, may be heard with a stethoscope partly off the chest (thrills are associated)
6/6 or VI/VI	may be heard with the stethoscope entirely off the chest (thrills are associated)

Apothecary symbols

The symbols presented below are for informational use. The apothecary system should *not* be used. Only the metric system should be used. The methods of expressing the symbols, the meanings, and the equivalences are not the classic ones, nor are they accurate, but reflect the usual intended meanings when used by some older physicians in writing prescription directions.

ʒ or ʒi̇	dram, teaspoonful, (5 mL)	℥ or ℥i̇	ounce, (30 mL)
ʒïï	two drams, 2 teaspoonfuls, (10 mL)	gr	grain (approximately 60 mg)
℥ss̄	half ounce, tablespoonful, (15 mL)	♏	minim (approximately 0.06 mL)
		gtt	drop

References

1. CBE Style Manual, 5th ed. Bethesda, MD: Council of Biology Editors; 1983.

2. Gennaro AR, ed. Remington's Pharmaceutical Sciences. 17th ed. Easton, PA: Mack Publishing Co; 1985; 1780.

3. Davis NM, Cohen MR. Medication errors: causes and prevention. Huntingdon Valley, PA: Neil M. Davis Associates; 1981.

4. Cohen MR. Medication error reports. Hosp Pharm (appears monthly from 1975 to the present).

5. Cohen MR. Medication errors. Nursing 90 (appears monthly, starting in Nursing 77, to the present).

6. Bates B. A guide to physical examinations. 4th ed. Philadelphia: J.B. Lippincott; 1987.

Please forward additional meanings for these abbreviations, additional abbreviations and their meanings, or corrections to the author so that the list can be updated. Thank you. **Dr. Neil M. Davis, 1143 Wright Drive, Huntingdon Valley, PA 19006. FAX (215) 938 1937**

Please forward additional meanings for these abbreviations, additional abbreviations and their meanings, or corrections to the author so that the list can be updated. Thank you. Dr. Neil M. Davis, 1143 Wright Drive, Huntingdon Valley, PA 19006.

Additions

PRICE

1-4 copies	**$9.95 each**	When check or money order *accompanies* the order. **If payment is not included, a $2.00 fee per order will be added to cover the cost of invoicing**
5-19 copies	**$9.95 each**	Purchase order accepted. No invoicing fee.
20 or more	**$7.10 each**	Purchase order accepted. No invoicing fee

United States—Postage cost is included in the price. Pennsylvania residents add 6% sales tax.

Outside the United States—Prices as shown above plus postage. Pay in U.S. dollars through a correspondent U.S. bank.

Order from

Neil M. Davis Associates
1143 Wright Drive
Huntingdon Valley, PA 19006
Phone (215) 947-1752
FAX (215) 938-1937

ISBN 0-931431-15-0

PROCARDIA XL® (nifedipine) Extended Release Tablets *For Oral Us*

DESCRIPTION: Nifedipine is a drug belonging to a class of pharmacological agents known as the calcium chann blockers. Nifedipine is 3,5-pyridinedicarboxylic acid, 1,4-dihydro-2,6-dimethyl-4-(2-nitrophenyl)-, dimethyl este $C_{17}H_{18}N_2O_6$.

Nifedipine is a yellow crystalline substance, practically insoluble in water but soluble in ethanol. It has a molecul weight of 346.3. PROCARDIA XL is a trademark for Nifedipine GITS. Nifedipine GITS (Gastrointestinal Therapeut System) Tablet is formulated as a once-a-day controlled-release tablet for oral administration designed to deliver 30, 6 or 90 mg of nifedipine.

Inert ingredients in the formulations are: cellulose acetate; hydroxypropyl cellulose; hydroxypropyl methylcellulos magnesium stearate; polyethylene glycol; polyethylene oxide; red ferric oxide; sodium chloride; titanium dioxide.

System Components and Performance: PROCARDIA XL Extended Release Tablet is similar in appearance to conventional tablet. It consists, however, of a semipermeable membrane surrounding an osmotically active drug cor The core itself is divided into two layers: an "active" layer containing the drug, and a "push" layer containin pharmacologically inert (but osmotically active) components. As water from the gastrointestinal tract enters the tabl pressure increases in the osmotic layer and "pushes" against the drug layer, releasing drug through the precision lase drilled tablet orifice in the active layer.

PROCARDIA XL Extended Release Tablet is designed to provide nifedipine at an approximately constant rate over 2 hours. This controlled rate of drug delivery into the gastrointestinal lumen is independent of pH or gastrointestin motility. PROCARDIA XL depends for its action on the existence of an osmotic gradient between the contents of the b layer core and fluid in the GI tract. Drug delivery is essentially constant as long as the osmotic gradient remains consta and then gradually falls to zero. Upon swallowing, the biologically inert components of the tablet remain intact during transit and are eliminated in the feces as an insoluble shell.

CLINICAL PHARMACOLOGY: Nifedipine is a calcium ion influx inhibitor (slow-channel blocker or calcium i antagonist) and inhibits the transmembrane influx of calcium ions into cardiac muscle and smooth muscle. T contractile processes of cardiac muscle and vascular smooth muscle are dependent upon the movement of extracellu calcium ions into these cells through specific ion channels. Nifedipine selectively inhibits calcium ion influx across t cell membrane of cardiac muscle and vascular smooth muscle without altering serum calcium concentrations.

Mechanism of Action:

A) Angina: The precise mechanisms by which inhibition of calcium influx relieves angina has not been fu determined, but includes at least the following two mechanisms:

1. Relaxation and Prevention of Coronary Artery Spasm: Nifedipine dilates the main coronary arteries and corona arterioles, both in normal and ischemic regions, and is a potent inhibitor of coronary artery spasm, whether spontaneo or ergonovine-induced. This property increases myocardial oxygen delivery in patients with coronary artery spasm, a is responsible for the effectiveness of nifedipine in vasospastic (Prinzmetal's or variant) angina. Whether this effect pla any role in classical angina is not clear, but studies of exercise tolerance have not shown an increase in the maximu exercise rate-pressure product, a widely accepted measure of oxygen utilization. This suggests that, in general, relief spasm or dilation of coronary arteries is not an important factor in classical angina.

2. Reduction of Oxygen Utilization: Nifedipine regularly reduces arterial pressure at rest and at a given level exercise by dilating peripheral arterioles and reducing the total peripheral vascular resistance (afterload) against whi the heart works. This unloading of the heart reduces myocardial energy consumption and oxygen requirements, a probably accounts for the effectiveness of nifedipine in chronic stable angina.

B) Hypertension: The mechanism by which nifedipine reduces arterial blood pressure involves peripheral arteri vasodilatation and the resulting reduction in peripheral vascular resistance. The increased peripheral vascular resistan that is an underlying cause of hypertension results from an increase in active tension in the vascular smooth muscl Studies have demonstrated that the increase in active tension reflects an increase in cytosolic free calcium.

Nifedipine is a peripheral arterial vasodilator which acts directly on vascular smooth muscle. The binding of nifedipin to voltage-dependent and possibly receptor-operated channels in vascular smooth muscle results in an inhibition o calcium influx through these channels. Stores of intracellular calcium in vascular smooth muscle are limited and thu dependent upon the influx of extracellular calcium for contraction to occur. The reduction in calcium influx by nifedipin causes arterial vasodilation and decreased peripheral vascular resistance which results in reduced arterial bloo pressure.

Pharmacokinetics and Metabolism: Nifedipine is completely absorbed after oral administration. Plasma drug concentrations rise at a gradual, controlled rate after a PROCARDIA XL Extended Release Tablet dose and reach a plateau at approximately six hours after the first dose. For subsequent doses, relatively constant plasma concentrations at this plateau are maintained with minimal fluctuations over the 24 hour dosing interval. About a four-fold higher fluctuation index (ratio of peak to trough plasma concentration) was observed with the conventional immediate release Procardia® capsule at t.i.d. dosing than with once daily PROCARDIA XL Extended Release Tablet. At steady-state the bioavailability of the PROCARDIA XL Extended Release Tablet is 86% relative to Procardia capsules. Administration of the PROCARDIA XL Extended Release Tablet in the presence of food slightly alters the early rate of drug absorption, but does not influence the extent of drug bioavailability. Markedly reduced GI retention time over prolonged periods (i.e., short bowel syndrome), however, may influence the pharmacokinetic profile of the drug which could potentially result in lower plasma concentrations. Pharmacokinetics of PROCARDIA XL Extended Release Tablets are linear over the dose range of 30 to 180 mg in that plasma drug concentrations are proportional to dose administered. There was no evidence of dose dumping either in the presence or absence of food for over 150 subjects in pharmacokinetic studies.

Nifedipine is extensively metabolized to highly water-soluble, inactive metabolites accounting for 60 to 80% of the dose excreted in the urine. The elimination half-life of nifedipine is approximately two hours. Only traces (less than 0.1% of the dose) of unchanged form can be detected in the urine. The remainder is excreted in the feces in metabolized form, most likely as a result of biliary excretion. Thus, the pharmacokinetics of nifedipine are not significantly influenced by the degree of renal impairment. Patients in hemodialysis or chronic ambulatory peritoneal dialysis have not reported significantly altered pharmacokinetics of nifedipine. Since hepatic biotransformation is the predominant route for the disposition of nifedipine, the pharmacokinetics may be altered in patients with chronic liver disease. Patients with hepatic impairment (liver cirrhosis) have a longer disposition half-life and higher bioavailability of nifedipine than healthy volunteers. The degree of serum protein binding of nifedipine is high (92-98%). Protein binding may be greatly reduced in patients with renal or hepatic impairment.

Hemodynamics: Like other slow-channel blockers, nifedipine exerts a negative inotropic effect on isolated myocardial tissue. This is rarely, if ever, seen in intact animals or man, probably because of reflex responses to its vasodilating effects. In man, nifedipine decreases peripheral vascular resistance which leads to a fall in systolic and diastolic pressures, usually minimal in normotensive volunteers (less than 5-10 mm Hg systolic), but sometimes larger. With PROCARDIA XL (nifedipine) Extended Release Tablets, these decreases in blood pressure are not accompanied by any significant change in heart rate. Hemodynamic studies in patients with normal ventricular function have generally found a small increase in cardiac index without major effects on ejection fraction, left ventricular end diastolic pressure (LVEDP) or volume (LVEDV). In patients with impaired ventricular function, most acute studies have shown some increase in ejection fraction and reduction in left ventricular filling pressure.

Electrophysiologic Effects: Although, like other members of its class, nifedipine causes a slight depression of sinoatrial node function and atrioventricular conduction in isolated myocardial preparations, such effects have not been seen in studies in intact animals or in man. In formal electrophysiologic studies, predominantly in patients with normal conduction systems, nifedipine has had no tendency to prolong atrioventricular conduction or sinus node recovery time, or to slow sinus rate.

INDICATIONS AND USAGE: **I. Vasospastic Angina:** PROCARDIA XL is indicated for the management of vasospastic angina confirmed by any of the following criteria: 1) classical pattern of angina at rest accompanied by ST segment elevation, 2) angina or coronary artery spasm provoked by ergonovine, or 3) angiographically demonstrated coronary artery spasm. In those patients who have had angiography, the presence of significant fixed obstructive disease is not incompatible with the diagnosis of vasospastic angina, provided that the above criteria are satisfied. PROCARDIA XL may also be used where the clinical presentation suggests a possible vasospastic component but where vasospasm has not been confirmed, e.g., where pain has a variable threshold on exertion or in unstable angina where electrocardiographic findings are compatible with intermittent vasospasm, or when angina is refractory to nitrates and/or adequate doses of beta blockers.

II. Chronic Stable Angina (Classical Effort-Associated Angina): PROCARDIA XL is indicated for the management of chronic stable angina (effort-associated angina) without evidence of vasospasm in patients who remain symptomatic despite adequate doses of beta blockers and/or organic nitrates or who cannot tolerate those agents.

In chronic stable angina (effort-associated angina) nifedipine has been effective in controlled trials of up to eight weeks duration in reducing angina frequency and increasing exercise tolerance, but confirmation of sustained effectiveness and evaluation of long term safety in these patients is incomplete.

Controlled studies in small numbers of patients suggest concomitant use of nifedipine and beta blocking agents may be beneficial in patients with chronic stable angina, but available information is not sufficient to predict with confidence the effects of concurrent treatment, especially in patients with compromised left ventricular function or cardiac conduction abnormalities. When introducing such concomitant therapy, care must be taken to monitor blood pressure closely since severe hypotension can occur from the combined effects of the drugs. (See WARNINGS.)

III. Hypertension: PROCARDIA XL is indicated for the treatment of hypertension. It may be used alone or in combination with other antihypertensive agents.

CONTRAINDICATIONS: Known hypersensitivity reaction to nifedipine.

WARNINGS: Excessive Hypotension: Although in most angina patients the hypotensive effect of nifedipine is modest and well tolerated, occasional patients have had excessive and poorly tolerated hypotension. These responses have usually occurred during initial titration or at the time of subsequent upward dosage adjustment, and may be more likely in patients on concomitant beta blockers.

Severe hypotension and/or increased fluid volume requirements have been reported in patients receiving nifedipine together with a beta-blocking agent who underwent coronary artery bypass surgery using high dose fentanyl anesthesia. The interaction with high dose fentanyl appears to be due to the combination of nifedipine and a beta blocker, but the possibility that it may occur with nifedipine alone, with low doses of fentanyl, in other surgical procedures, or with other narcotic analgesics cannot be ruled out. In nifedipine-treated patients where surgery using high dose fentanyl anesthesia is contemplated, the physician should be aware of these potential problems and if the patient's condition permits, sufficient time (at least 36 hours) should be allowed for nifedipine to be washed out of the body prior to surgery.

The following information should be taken into account in those patients who are being treated for hypertension as well as angina:

Increased Angina and/or Myocardial Infarction: Rarely, patients, particularly those who have severe obstructive coronary artery disease, have developed well documented increased frequency, duration and/or severity of angina or acute myocardial infarction on starting nifedipine or at the time of dosage increase. The mechanism of this effect is not established.

Beta Blocker Withdrawal: It is important to taper beta blockers if possible, rather than stopping them abruptly before beginning nifedipine. Patients recently withdrawn from beta blockers may develop a withdrawal syndrome with increased angina, probably related to increased sensitivity to catecholamines. Initiation of nifedipine treatment will not prevent this occurrence and on occasion has been reported to increase it.

Congestive Heart Failure: Rarely, patients usually receiving a beta blocker, have developed heart failure after beginning nifedipine. Patients with tight aortic stenosis may be at greater risk for such an event, as the unloading effect of nifedipine would be expected to be of less benefit to those patients, owing to their fixed impedance to flow across the aortic valve.

PRECAUTIONS: General—Hypotension: Because nifedipine decreases peripheral vascular resistance, careful monitoring of blood pressure during the initial administration and titration of nifedipine is suggested. Close observation is especially recommended for patients already taking medications that are known to lower blood pressure. (See WARNINGS.)

Peripheral Edema: Mild to moderate peripheral edema occurs in a dose dependent manner with an incidence ranging from approximately 10% to about 30% at the highest dose studied (180 mg). It is a localized phenomenon thought to be associated with vasodilation of dependent arterioles and small blood vessels and not due to left ventricular dysfunction or generalized fluid retention. With patients whose angina or hypertension is complicated by congestive heart failure, care should be taken to differentiate this peripheral edema from the effects of increasing left ventricular dysfunction.

Other: As with any other non-deformable material, caution should be used when administering PROCARDIA XL in patients with preexisting severe gastrointestinal narrowing (pathologic or iatrogenic). There have been rare reports of obstructive symptoms in patients with known strictures in association with the ingestion of PROCARDIA XL.

Information for Patients: PROCARDIA XL® (nifedipine) Extended Release Tablets should be swallowed whole. Do not chew, divide or crush tablets. Do not be concerned if you occasionally notice in your stool something that looks like a tablet. In PROCARDIA XL, the medication is contained within a nonabsorbable shell that has been specially designed to slowly release the drug for your body to absorb. When this process is completed, the empty tablet is eliminated from your body.

Laboratory Tests: Rare, usually transient, but occasionally significant elevations of enzymes such as alkaline phosphatase, CPK, LDH, SGOT, and SGPT have been noted. The relationship to nifedipine therapy is uncertain in most cases, but probable in some. These laboratory abnormalities have rarely been associated with clinical symptoms: however, cholestasis with or without jaundice has been reported. A small (5.4%) increase in mean alkaline phosphatase was noted in patients treated with PROCARDIA XL. This was an isolated finding not associated with clinical symptoms and it rarely resulted in values which fell outside the normal range. Rare instances of allergic hepatitis have been reported. In controlled studies, PROCARDIA XL did not adversely affect serum uric acid, glucose, or cholesterol. Serum potassium was unchanged in patients receiving PROCARDIA XL in the absence of concomitant diuretic therapy, and slightly decreased in patients receiving concomitant diuretics.

Nifedipine, like other calcium channel blockers, decreases platelet aggregation *in vitro*. Limited clinical studies have demonstrated a moderate but statistically significant decrease in platelet aggregation and increase in bleeding time in some nifedipine patients. This is thought to be a function of inhibition of calcium transport across the platelet membrane. No clinical significance for these findings has been demonstrated.

Positive direct Coombs test with/without hemolytic anemia has been reported but a causal relationship between nifedipine administration and positivity of this laboratory test, including hemolysis, could not be determined.

Although nifedipine has been used safely in patients with renal dysfunction and has been reported to exert a beneficial effect in certain cases, rare reversible elevations in BUN and serum creatinine have been reported in patients with pre-existing chronic renal insufficiency. The relationship to nifedipine therapy is uncertain in most cases but probable in some.

Drug Interactions: Beta-adrenergic blocking agents: (See INDICATIONS AND WARNINGS) Experience in over 1400 patients with Procardia capsules in a noncomparative clinical trial has shown that concomitant administration of nifedipine and beta-blocking agents is usually well tolerated but there have been occasional literature reports suggesting that the combination may increase the likelihood of congestive heart failure, severe hypotension, or exacerbation of angina.

Long Acting Nitrates: Nifedipine may be safely co-administered with nitrates, but there have been no controlled studies to evaluate the antianginal effectiveness of this combination.

Digitalis: Administration of nifedipine with digoxin increased digoxin levels in nine of twelve normal volunteers. The average increase was 45%. Another investigator found no increase in digoxin levels in thirteen patients with coronary artery disease. In an uncontrolled study of over two hundred patients with congestive heart failure during which digoxin blood levels were not measured, digitalis toxicity was not observed. Since there have been isolated reports of patients with elevated digoxin levels, it is recommended that digoxin levels be monitored when initiating, adjusting, and discontinuing nifedipine to avoid possible over- or under-digitalization.

Coumarin Anticoagulants: There have been rare reports of increased prothrombin time in patients taking coumarin anticoagulants to whom nifedipine was administered. However, the relationship to nifedipine therapy is uncertain.

Cimetidine: A study in six healthy volunteers has shown a significant increase in peak nifedipine plasma levels (80%) and area-under-the-curve (74%), after a one week course of cimetidine at 1000 mg per day and nifedipine at 40 mg per day. Ranitidine produced smaller, non-significant increases. The effect may be mediated by the known inhibition of cimetidine on hepatic cytochrome P-450, the enzyme system probably responsible for the first-pass metabolism of nifedipine. If nifedipine therapy is initiated in a patient currently receiving cimetidine, cautious titration is advised.

Carcinogenesis, Mutagenesis, Impairment of Fertility: Nifedipine was administered orally to rats for two years and was not shown to be carcinogenic. When given to rats prior to mating, nifedipine caused reduced fertility at a dose approximately 30 times the maximum recommended human dose. *In vivo* mutagenicity studies were negative.

Pregnancy: Pregnancy Category C. Nifedipine has been shown to be teratogenic in rats when given in doses 30 times the maximum recommended human dose. Nifedipine was embryotoxic (increased fetal resorptions, decreased fetal weight, increased stunted forms, increased fetal deaths, decreased neonatal survival) in rats, mice, and rabbits at doses of from 3 to 10 times the maximum recommended human dose. In pregnant monkeys, doses 2/3 and twice the maximum recommended human dose resulted in small placentas and underdeveloped chorionic villi. In rats, doses three times maximum human dose and higher caused prolongation of pregnancy. There are no adequate and well controlled studies in pregnant women. PROCARDIA XL Extended Release Tablets should be used during pregnancy only if the potential benefit justifies the potential risk to the fetus.

ADVERSE EXPERIENCES: Over 1000 patients from both controlled and open trials with PROCARDIA XL Extended Release Tablets in hypertension and angina were included in the evaluation of adverse experiences. All side effects reported during PROCARDIA XL Extended Release Tablet therapy were tabulated independent of their causal relation to medication. The most common side effect reported with PROCARDIA XL was edema which was dose related and ranged in frequency from approximately 10% to about 30% at the highest dose studied (180 mg). Other common adverse experiences reported in placebo-controlled trials include:

Adverse Effect	**PROCARDIA XL (%) (N=707)**	**Placebo (%) (N=266)**
Headache	15.8	9.8
Fatigue	5.9	4.1
Dizziness	4.1	4.5
Constipation	3.3	2.3
Nausea	3.3	1.9

Of these, only edema and headache were more common in PROCARDIA XL patients than placebo patients.

The following adverse reactions occurred with an incidence of less than 3.0%. With the exception of leg cramps, the incidence of these side effects was similar to that of placebo alone.

Body as a Whole/Systemic: asthenia, flushing, pain
Cardiovascular: palpitations
Central Nervous System: insomnia, nervousness, paresthesia, somnolence
Dermatologic: pruritus, rash
Gastrointestinal: abdominal pain, diarrhea, dry mouth, dyspepsia, flatulence
Musculoskeletal: arthralgia, leg cramps
Respiratory: chest pain (nonspecific), dyspnea
Urogenital: impotence, polyuria

Other adverse reactions were reported sporadically with an incidence of 1.0% or less. These include:
Body as a Whole/Systemic: face edema, fever, hot flashes, malaise, periorbital edema, rigors
Cardiovascular: arrhythmia, hypotension, increased angina, tachycardia, syncope
Central Nervous System: anxiety, ataxia, decreased libido, depression, hypertonia, hypoesthesia, migraine, paroniria, tremor, vertigo
Dermatologic: alopecia, increased sweating, urticaria, purpura
Gastrointestinal: eructation, gastroesophageal reflux, gum hyperplasia, melena, vomiting, weight increase
Musculoskeletal: back pain, gout, myalgias
Respiratory: coughing, epistaxis, upper respiratory tract infection, respiratory disorder, sinusitis
Special Senses: abnormal lacrimation, abnormal vision, taste perversion, tinnitus
Urogenital/Reproductive: breast pain, dysuria, hematuria, nocturia

Adverse experiences which occurred in less than 1 in 1000 patients cannot be distinguished from concurrent disease states or medications.

The following adverse experiences, reported in less than 1% of patients, occurred under conditions (e.g. open trials, marketing experience) where a causal relationship is uncertain: gastrointestinal irritation, gastrointestinal bleeding.

In multiple-dose U.S. and foreign controlled studies with nifedipine capsules in which adverse reactions were reported spontaneously, adverse effects were frequent but generally not serious and rarely required discontinuation of therapy or dosage adjustment. Most were expected consequences of the vasodilator effects of Procardia.

Adverse Effect	**PROCARDIA CAPSULES (%) (N=226)**	**Placebo (%) (N=235)**
Dizziness, lightheadedness, giddiness	27	15
Flushing, heat sensation	25	8
Headache	23	20
Weakness	12	10
Nausea, heartburn	11	8
Muscle cramps, tremor	8	3
Peripheral edema	7	1
Nervousness, mood changes	7	4
Palpitation	7	5
Dyspnea, cough, wheezing	6	3
Nasal congestion, sore throat	6	8

There is also a large uncontrolled experience in over 2100 patients in the United States. Most of the patients had vasospastic or resistant angina pectoris, and about half had concomitant treatment with beta-adrenergic blocking agents. The relatively common adverse events were similar in nature to those seen with PROCARDIA XL® (nifedipine).

In addition, more serious adverse events were observed, not readily distinguishable from the natural history of the disease in these patients. It remains possible, however, that some or many of these events were drug related. Myocardial infarction occurred in about 4% of patients and congestive heart failure or pulmonary edema in about 2%. Ventricular arrhythmias or conduction disturbances each occurred in fewer than 0.5% of patients.

In a subgroup of over 1000 patients receiving Procardia with concomitant beta blocker therapy, the pattern and incidence of adverse experiences was not different from that of the entire group of Procardia treated patients (See PRECAUTIONS.)

In a subgroup of approximately 250 patients with a diagnosis of congestive heart failure as well as angina, dizziness or lightheadedness, peripheral edema, headache or flushing each occurred in one in eight patients. Hypotension occurred in about one in 20 patients. Syncope occurred in approximately one patient in 250. Myocardial infarction or symptoms of congestive heart failure each occurred in about one patient in 15. Atrial or ventricular dysrhythmias each occurred in about one patient in 150.

In post-marketing experience, there have been rare reports of exfoliative dermatitis caused by nifedipine.

OVERDOSAGE: Experience with nifedipine overdosage is limited. Generally, overdosage with nifedipine leading to pronounced hypotension calls for active cardiovascular support including monitoring of cardiovascular and respiratory function, elevation of extremities, judicious use of calcium infusion, pressor agents and fluids. Clearance of nifedipine would be expected to be prolonged in patients with impaired liver function. Since nifedipine is highly protein-bound, dialysis is not likely to be of any benefit.

There has been one reported case of massive overdosage with PROCARDIA XL Extended Release Tablets. The main effects of ingestion of approximately 4800 mg of PROCARDIA XL in a young man attempting suicide as a result of cocaine-induced depression was initial dizziness, palpitations, flushing, and nervousness. Within several hours of ingestion, nausea, vomiting, and generalized edema developed. No significant hypotension was apparent at presentation, 18 hours post-ingestion. Electrolyte abnormalities consisted of a mild, transient elevation of serum creatinine, and modest elevations of LDH and CPK, but normal SGOT. Vital signs remained stable, no electrocardiographic abnormalities were noted and renal function returned to normal within 24 to 48 hours with routine supportive measures alone. No prolonged sequelae were observed.

The effect of a single 900 mg ingestion of Procardia capsules in a depressed anginal patient also on tricyclic antidepressants was loss of consciousness within 30 minutes of ingestion, and profound hypotension, which responded to calcium infusion, pressor agents, and fluid replacement. A variety of ECG abnormalities were seen in this patient with a history of bundle branch block, including sinus bradycardia and varying degrees of AV block. These dictated the prophylactic placement of a temporary ventricular pacemaker, but otherwise resolved spontaneously. Significant hyperglycemia was seen initially in this patient, but plasma glucose levels rapidly normalized without further treatment.

A young hypertensive patient with advanced renal failure ingested 280 mg of Procardia capsules at one time, with resulting marked hypotension responding to calcium infusion and fluids. No AV conduction abnormalities, arrhythmias, or pronounced changes in heart rate were noted, nor was there any further deterioration in renal function.

DOSAGE AND ADMINISTRATION: Dosage must be adjusted according to each patient's needs. Therapy for either hypertension or angina should be initiated with 30 or 60 mg once daily. PROCARDIA XL® (nifedipine) Extended Release Tablets should be swallowed whole and should not be bitten or divided. In general, titration should proceed over a 7-14 day period so that the physician can fully assess the response to each dose level and monitor blood pressure before proceeding to higher doses. Since steady-state plasma levels are achieved on the second day of dosing, if symptoms so warrant, titration may proceed more rapidly provided the patient is assessed frequently. Titration to doses above 120 mg are not recommended.

Angina patients controlled on Procardia capsules alone or in combination with other antianginal medications may be safely switched to PROCARDIA XL Extended Release Tablets at the nearest equivalent total daily dose (e.g. 30 mg t.i.d. of Procardia capsules may be changed to 90 mg once daily of PROCARDIA XL Extended Release Tablets). Subsequent titration to higher or lower doses may be necessary and should be initiated as clinically warranted. Experience with doses greater than 90 mg in patients with angina is limited. Therefore, doses greater than 90 mg should be used with caution and only when clinically warranted.

No "rebound effect" has been observed upon discontinuation of PROCARDIA XL Extended Release Tablets. However, if discontinuation of nifedipine is necessary, sound clinical practice suggests that the dosage should be decreased gradually with close physician supervision.

Care should be taken when dispensing PROCARDIA XL to assure that the extended release dosage form has been prescribed.

Co-Administration with Other Antianginal Drugs: Sublingual nitroglycerin may be taken as required for the control of acute manifestations of angina, particularly during nifedipine titration. See PRECAUTIONS, Drug Interactions, for information on co-administration of nifedipine with beta blockers or long acting nitrates.

HOW SUPPLIED: PROCARDIA XL Extended Release Tablets are supplied as 30 mg, 60 mg and 90 mg round biconvex, rose-pink, film-coated tablets in

Bottles of 100: 30 mg (NDC 0069-2650-66); 60 mg (NDC 0069-2660-66); 90 mg (NDC 0069-2670-66)
Bottles of 300: 30 mg (NDC 0069-2650-72); 60 mg (NDC 0069-2660-72)
Unit dose packages of 100: 30 mg (NDC 0069-2650-41); 60 mg (NDC 0069-2660-41)
The tablets should be protected from moisture and humidity and stored below 86°F (30°C).

Revised July 1990